D1481451

Children with Osteogenesis Imperfecta: Strategies to Enhance Performance

Holly Lea Cintas, PT, PhD, and Lynn H. Gerber, MD

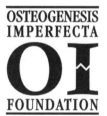

OSTEOGENESIS IMPERFECTA

OI

FOUNDATION

Osteogenesis Imperfecta Foundation, Inc.
Gaithersburg, Maryland

Osteogenesis Imperfecta Foundation, Inc.
804 West Diamond Avenue, Suite 210
Gaithersburg, MD 20878

ISBN 0-9642189-5-X

ISBN 0-9642189-5-X

5 1 0 0 0

9 780964 218956

Contents

(continued)

Foreword

A lot has changed in the osteogenesis imperfecta community. Not so long ago parents were advised to carry their child on a pillow; and children and adults were told to avoid movement and most recreational activities. Now, based on information from years of clinical experience, a better approach is available. Instead of immobilization, increased physical activity and exercise, and a wider range of therapeutic and recreational activities, are recommended.

Research indicates that being physically active has many benefits. It improves general health through cardiovascular fitness, increased mental alertness, and weight control. Physical activity also promotes maximal bone density and bone growth. It improves self-confidence and allows the development of skills that lead to greater independence in day-to-day living. Although muscle weakness, joint stiffness or laxity, low stamina, and of course, fragile bones are realities that need to be addressed, the bottom line is that making the effort to be more physically active is worth it.

The first year of life is a window of opportunity to help babies develop their ability to move. Childhood and the teen years are a time to learn and refine skills, develop strength, and have fun. Adults are encouraged to follow a healthy, active life style. Although physical activity and exercise will not cure osteogenesis imperfecta, they will help improve the quality of life and health of each individual. Participation can help build healthier bodies, minds, and spirits.

Because there is a high degree of variation among people who have osteogenesis imperfecta, it is not possible to suggest a single, detailed fitness plan that will work for everyone. Activities must be carefully chosen and adapted to the individual's age, abilities, goals, and interests. This book is intended as a guide for parents, teens, and healthcare providers. It suggests recreational activities, intervention strategies, adaptive equipment, and resources for a wide range of needs and ages.

It is never too late for adults, older children, and teens to make a habit of exercise. Increasing physical activity means starting from where you are right now and doing a little more. Enjoyment plus improved function will be the end result.

I'm pleased to be able to share my personal story with you as an example of how exercise can improve your mobility and your outlook. Whether you are trying to transfer from wheelchair to bed, or run a mile, you can benefit from exercise. I hope that my personal story, and the ideas in this book, can inspire you to start moving and have fun in the process!

One of the best ways I've found to stay strong and healthy with OI is through exercise. Staying active has always been very important for my family. When I was in grade school, my brother was busy all year playing football, basketball, and baseball. At that time, there were no local adapted recreation/sports programs for me to get my exercise in the same structured way. I'm thankful that my family was creative in finding outlets for my own quite large supply of energy. During my brother's practices, I often walked around a nearby track using my walker. Sometimes I would push my wheelchair around the tennis court to build up endurance. The important thing was that, like my brother, I had a routine and a schedule for my exercise. This way, I was able to see improvement, set goals, and get stronger. In highschool, I remained active in sports and decided to try wheelchair track. I trained with my school's track team. Whatever distance they did, I could usually divide that in half and finish in the same amount of time. With the help of patient coaches and some creativity, we worked on my starts and on different strategies I could use during my own races. I entered 5K races in the area and tried to better my times each weekend. I was almost always the only entrant in the wheelchair division, but whether I "won" or not depended on whether I had improved my time. I looked forward to attending Wright State University as my college of choice because I knew they had an excellent adapted sports program. Little did I know my wheelchair track days would definitely be coming to an end!

My freshman year at Wright State was so exciting. It was the first time I was able to participate in a sports program for people with disabilities. I took an adapted fitness class my first semester and designed a workout that would be safe and effective for me. Five years later, I still use much of it (with a few tweaks). I am able to build muscle by using small weights and more repetitions. Stretching is important before lifting as a way to get my body loose and ready to work. I get out of my chair for this and use a mat. I've found floor work has helped me get stronger in many ways. I do leg lifts and raises to strengthen my legs and hip muscles. My hips can become pretty contracted from sitting so much. It's important to keep them strong so they can keep my body in a straight line. In the gym, I'm also able to use the rowing machine and the hand cycle. Both are great ways to build cardiovascular endurance. I also got in shape my first year of college by playing many of the intramural sports offered for people with disabilities. I played handball, tennis, Frisbee golf, and even wheelchair football. It's safer than you'd think!

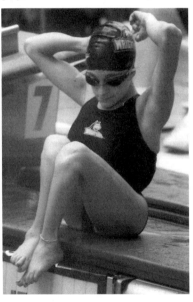

All this activity was a fun way to get exercise and meet new people. I discovered that wheelchair track wasn't really for me, and I found a sport that I loved even more, swimming. I had always loved the water, swimming with my cousins, working at the pool during the summers, playing in the Kentucky River, and using the pool as a place to heal after fractures. I guess it should have been obvious that this sport was going to be a good fit for me. I started learning proper strokes and working on my techniques. After my very first season, I qualified for the Disability National Championships for backstroke. I did okay at that meet, but definitely had room for improvement. During my second year, I started training every day and my times dropped steadily. I set my first American and world records that summer. Four years later, I would be the only person with osteogenesis imperfecta to represent the United States in the 2004 Paralympic Games in Athens, Greece. It's amazing how far exercise and hard work can take you!

Of course, along the road, there are always unexpected detours. Living with OI, I'm practiced at adapting, but I can't say I ever get used to it. I've had a few fractures and several tissue strains or tears that have caused me to take time out of the water. Different kinds of exercise have helped me heal more quickly and hold onto the strength I work so hard to maintain. Resistance cords for the parts that are not injured are low impact tools that can help stretch and strengthen arms and legs. I've also learned exercises from trainers to strengthen my weaker areas to prevent future injuries. For me, I have to keep my legs and hips moving both in and out of the water. I've also had to set my priorities and work hard to stay healthy for swimming. Of course, I'm always careful to a point, but during swim season, I try to refrain from doing other activities that put unnecessary strain on my shoulders. I've also learned to speak up if someone asks me to do something or suggests an exercise or sport that isn't safe for me. Part of exercising is staying healthy so you are able to do it. Sometimes it's difficult, but setting priorities will help you in many areas of life. For me, I definitely had to retire from my days as a wheelchair football quarterback!

For every sacrifice, I've been given so many gifts from my participation in sports and exercise activities. I've stayed stronger, learned to balance my time, and stayed on top of my schoolwork. I've learned to travel, often alone, to go to meets and compete. I'm able to transfer more safely and quickly. I can feel a difference in my body if I take even a few days off from some form of exercise. I'm very thankful for the independence that swimming and exercise have given me. Setting my goals to be faster and stronger keeps me going, even on those days when I'd rather just lounge. Another motivation for me is all of the friendships I've made, and interesting people I've met along the way. Once I was fortunate enough to have a team, I learned how that bond can get you through some challenging workouts. I love meeting other competitors with disabilities across the world. This summer, I met other people with osteogenesis imperfecta from New Zealand, England, and Jamaica. We are all proud to have overcome our fractures and now use our strong bodies to compete for our countries.

The experience of living with osteogenesis imperfecta has been one of pain and joy for me. The joy of reaching my goals and connecting with others keeps me going and the pain reminds me that there's really nothing I can't do. We've all recovered from several fractures, surgeries, and some pretty brutal physical therapy sessions. Exercise is another way to reach your dreams, whatever they may be. So, when someone says, "Feel the burn!" just use those strengths you already have as a proud person with OI. Get out there and do something!

Kara Sheridan

World record holder, 200-meter breaststroke, SB4 classification

American record holder, 50-, 100-, and 200-meter breaststroke

American record holder, 100-meter backstroke

Paralympic athlete, 2004

Team USA member, Paralympic World Cup, Manchester, England, 2005

Ranked 1st in USA/9th in world, 100-meter breaststroke, as of May 2005

Ranked 4th in USA/23rd in world, 100-meter backstroke, as of June 2004

Sponsored by Challenged Athletes Foundation

BS in psychology and rehabilitation services, Wright State University

Acknowledgments

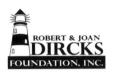

The Osteogenesis Imperfecta Foundation gratefully acknowledges the **Robert and Joan Dircks Foundation, Inc.** for generous funding to produce this book. Financial support from the foundation allowed the Osteogenesis Imperfecta Foundation to recruit volunteer editors Lynn H. Gerber, MD, and Holly Lea Cintas, PT, PhD, who contributed their combined 35 years of clinical experience to this book and recruited some of the best rehabilitation therapists working today for specific chapters. Additional support from the **GM Asian Indian Association** helped to expand the book's distribution to those who will benefit most.

No project this large could be accomplished without the help of many, many people who shared their time and talents with the Osteogenesis Imperfecta Foundation. The authors generously gave their time to write these high-quality chapters, distilling their years of clinical experience into specific recommendations for people with osteogenesis imperfecta. Most of the information included has not been published previously. Rather than having to spend hours in the library, searching the Internet, networking among support groups, or visiting numerous rehabilitation specialists, families are provided the valuable information shared by these experts in a readable and concise format. By contributing to this book, each author has truly made a difference in the lives of people living with osteogenesis imperfecta.

As each chapter was completed, volunteer occupational and physical therapists, parents of children with osteogenesis imperfecta, adults with the condition, rehabilitation physicians, orthopedic surgeons, and pediatricians read each chapter draft carefully, pointing out everything from missing commas to missing information. Their constructive criticism and praise helped the authors refine their drafts and craft each chapter into a practical and well-rounded resource. In addition to Osteogenesis Imperfecta Foundation staff members, the review committee included Helga Binder, MD; Jane Forbes, PT;

Michael Johnston; Marilyn King, OTR/L; Patricia Kipperman, OT; Bonnie Landrum, MD; Joan Marini, MD, Ph.D; Peter Smith, MD; and Meg Stanger, PT.

Following the reviews, Dr. Gerber and Dr. Cintas worked with each author to refine his or her chapter, then thoroughly reread every chapter at each stage to ensure accuracy and further clarify how the information is presented. In addition, they combed through their photo files to come up with illustrative photos to help explain concepts and show strategies and practical suggestions that can help children perform desired (and necessary) activities. It is interesting to note that the majority of these photos show children who are smiling and enjoying what they are doing. We are grateful to the many families who contributed photos to this valuable book. They have given all of us a tremendous resource.

Osteogenesis Imperfecta Foundation staff members provided vital support to this project. Mary Beth Huber brought to bear her experience providing information to adults and to families and their children with osteogenesis imperfecta; her insights on what information families need and how it should be presented were invaluable. She also painstakingly verified the accuracy of Web sites and equipment information, with the assistance of Marie Maffey. William Bradner assisted with the design and printing process, ensuring a quality product. Erika Ruebensaal developed promotional materials that will help the book find a wide audience. Consulting Editor Heidi Green arrived at a critical time to help with the technical aspects of editing.

As I read each draft of the book, I shared what I was learning with families across the country, all of whom are now eagerly awaiting publication. It has been, and will continue to be, an honor to offer this invaluable resource to people with osteogenesis imperfecta of all ages who want to enhance their capabilities and improve their quality of life. We at the Osteogenesis Imperfecta Foundation are extremely proud to support the dissemination of this practical information to help promote health, hope, and happiness for all people with osteogenesis imperfecta.

Heller An Shapiro
Executive Director

Contributors

Holly Lea Cintas, PT, PhD

Dr. Cintas is Physical Therapy Research Coordinator, Rehabilitation Medicine Department, at the National Institutes of Health (NIH). She has a BS in physical therapy from the University of Colorado and a PhD in developmental psychology from the University of Pennsylvania. Prior to coming to the NIH, Dr. Cintas was Associate Professor of Physical Therapy at Thomas Jefferson University, where she received the Lindback Award for Excellence in Teaching. Dr. Cintas has served as Inpatient Supervisor at Children's Hospital, Boston, and Director of Physical Therapy at Children's Hospital of Philadelphia. She is board certified in pediatric physical therapy, coauthor of the *Handbook of Pediatric Physical Therapy* (1st Edition), and former president of the Section on Pediatrics of the American Physical Therapy Association. She currently serves on the Board of Directors of the American Academy of Cerebral Palsy and Developmental Medicine and on the Medical Advisory Council of the Osteogenesis Imperfecta Foundation. She is a frequent presenter at Osteogenesis Imperfecta Foundation national conferences and is the coauthor of the chapter "Exercise and Activity: A Balance Between Work and Play" in *Growing Up with OI: A Guide for Families and Caregivers*. Her research interests have included the origins of fetal movement and cross-cultural variations in motor behavior. Her current research emphasis is the assessment of nonkinetic influences on motor development and their relationship to motor performance in children with osteogenesis imperfecta. She is the mother of a son and a daughter.

Lynn H. Gerber, MD

Dr. Gerber is Chief, Rehabilitation Medicine Department, at the NIH. In this capacity she assures the quality of physical medicine and rehabilitation evaluations and treatments for all referred NIH patients with impairments and disability. She also assures the quality and timeliness of research support and collaboration for NIH investigators by providing standardized treatment and devising, selecting, and administering functional outcome measures. The Rehabilitation Medicine Department also performs research on human movement as a joint effort with the National Institute of Child Health and Human Development. Dr. Gerber is on the staff of the National Rehabilitation Hospital and runs a teaching clinic on foot management as part of a bilateral agreement between the NIH and the hospital. Dr. Gerber is board certified in internal medicine, rheumatology, and physical medicine and rehabilitation. Much of her clinical research interest has been centered on measuring and treating impairments and disability in patients with musculoskeletal deficits; in particular, children with osteogenesis imperfecta, and persons with rheumatoid arthritis and cancer. She is a frequent presenter at Osteogenesis Imperfecta Foundation national conferences. Her collaborative work has been learning about pathomechanics and how patients with a variety of disorders compensate for impairments to preserve function. Dr. Gerber is the author or coauthor of 90 peer-reviewed published manuscripts and 45 chapters in major textbooks on internal medicine, rheumatology, cancer, and rehabilitation. She is the coauthor of the chapter "Exercise and Activity: A Balance Between Work and Play" in *Growing Up with OI: A Guide for Families and Caregivers*. Dr. Gerber is the mother of two daughters.

Scott M. Paul, MD

Dr. Paul is Research Coordinator for the Medical Staff Section of the Rehabilitation Medicine Department at the NIH. He received a Bachelor's of Engineering Science in bioengineering at the Johns Hopkins University and an MD at the Sackler School of Medicine of Tel Aviv University in Israel. Dr. Paul completed his postgraduate medical training at Washington University in St. Louis, Albert Einstein College of Medicine, and the Rose F. Kennedy Children's Evaluation and Treatment Center. He is board certified in physical medicine and rehabilitation and pediatric rehabilitation. Prior to joining the Rehabilitation Medicine Department at the NIH, Dr. Paul was in private practice in Montgomery County, Maryland, with Rehabilitation Medical Director responsibilities at Montgomery General, Shady Grove Adventist, and Gladys Spellman Specialty Hospitals. He previously served as Chief of Physical Medicine at Dayton Children's Medical Center and Director of Physical Medicine and Rehabilitation at the Hospital for Sick Children in Washington, DC. In addition to serving as an investigator in the NIH's osteogenesis imperfecta protocols, he participates in clinical research protocols related to polyostotic fibrous dysplasia, neonatal-onset multisystem inflammatory disease, Friedreich's ataxia, and neurofibromatosis. Dr. Paul wrote the chapter "Scoliosis and Other Spinal Deformities" in the newest edition of *Physical Medicine and Rehabilitation: Principles and Practice*. He is the author of numerous abstracts and articles on childhood-onset disabilities, including osteogenesis imperfecta. He is a presenter at Osteogenesis Imperfecta Foundation national conferences. Dr. Paul is the father of four children, three of whom are adolescents.

Maureen Donohoe, PT, DPT, PCS

Ms. Donohoe practices at the Alfred I. DuPont Hospital for Children. Her emphasis of care for more than 15 years has been pediatric orthopedic physical therapy. She received a BS in physical therapy from Thomas Jefferson University, Philadelphia, and has recently been enrolled at Simmons College in Boston for the Doctor of Physical Therapy degree. Her special interest is improving function for children who have osteogenesis imperfecta. She has had the opportunity to coauthor several book chapters on physical therapy management for children with osteogenesis imperfecta. She has also given local and international lectures on maximizing function for children with osteogenesis imperfecta. Although she has been working with children with osteogenesis imperfecta for more than 15 years, the true reality of safe infant handling occurred with the birth of her daughter in 2000.

Joanne Ruck-Gibis, PT, MSc

Ms. Ruck-Gibis has been Head of the Physiotherapy Department at the Shriners Hospital for Children in Montreal since 1988. She received a BSc in physiotherapy in 1976 and an MSc in rehabilitation from McGill University in 1999. Her master's projects included designing a booklet for families titled *Sports and Exercise for Children with OI* and writing "The Reliability of the Gross Motor Function Measure for Children with Osteogenesis Imperfecta" for the journal *Pediatric Physical Therapy* (2001). She obtained a Graduate Diploma in Institutional Administration from Concordia University in 1992, and is currently a part-time faculty lecturer at the School of Physical and Occupational Therapy at McGill. As a member of the interdisciplinary osteogenesis imperfecta clinic, her specific interests include the rehabilitation of children with osteogenesis imperfecta and functional outcomes following intramedullary rodding. She has had the opportunity to lecture on these topics in Lima, Peru; Dallas, Texas; Victoria, British Columbia; and Montreal, Quebec. She has also collaborated on a book titled *Interdisciplinary Treatment Approach for Children with Osteogenesis Imperfecta 2004*, and has participated in several studies at Shriners Hospital related to the treatment of osteogenesis imperfecta. Her other interests and areas of expertise include the transition of young adults with physical disabilities into the adult world and spasticity management in children with cerebral palsy, in relation to selective dorsal rhizotomy. She is the mother of a son.

Kathleen Malone Montpetit, OT, MSc

Ms. Malone Montpetit has been working at Shriners Hospital in Montreal since 1979 and is currently the Head of the Occupational Therapy Department and Outcomes Coordinator. She has a BSc in occupational therapy and a master's degree in rehabilitation from McGill University. She has been involved with the multidisciplinary osteogenesis imperfecta team of the Shriners Hospital Canadian Unit since its inception in 1995. She is the coauthor of several papers related to osteogenesis imperfecta, including a recent contribution to a new book on the multidisciplinary treatment of osteogenesis imperfecta. She is particularly interested in seating and mobility interventions available for children with osteogenesis imperfecta and the functional outcomes associated with early adaptive seating. She has given presentations at several international conferences on seating, mobility, and self-care strategies for children with osteogenesis imperfecta. Her professional interests include all seating and mobility interventions, and the integration of outcome tools into clinical practice. She is the mother of two daughters and a son.

Timothy J. Caruso, PT, MBA, MS

Mr. Caruso is a physical therapist whose 23 years of experience in healthcare have included home health, rehabilitation, thermal injuries, orthopedics, education, research, and pediatrics. He received his BS in physical therapy from Washington University in St Louis, and master's degrees in business administration and management from Benedictine University in Lisle, Illinois. Mr. Caruso has focused his professional expertise on manual therapy and orthopedics, specifically neuromusculoskeletal disorders. As founder of Chicagoland Performance Consultants, he currently works with industrial and professional organizations in the areas of management, job analysis, organizational dynamics, wellness, and injury prevention. He has worked as an educational consultant for Formations in Healthcare, a division of Medi-Risk Inc., training organizations and developing medical outcome instruments. He also provides direct patient care at Shriners Hospital for Children in Chicago and in his private practice. He sees children and adults with special needs for assessment, selection, and fitting of adaptive equipment and customized seating systems. He continues as a clinical instructor for physical therapy students at Shriners Hospital in Chicago and as an adjunct faculty member at the University of Illinois at the Chicago Program in Physical Therapy. He chairs the Ergonomics Committee at Shriners Hospital in Chicago and is developing a research project to determine the number of visits required for young children with special needs to learn to drive a power wheelchair. He is the father of two daughters.

CHAPTER ONE

INTRODUCTION

*The impact of osteogenesis imperfecta
on the musculoskeletal system
and its structural and functional
consequences*

Lynn H. Gerber, MD

O steogenesis imperfecta is a genetic disorder in which collagen, the most prevalent protein in the body, is abnormal in structure or deficient in quantity or both. The expression of the disorder varies widely with regard to which organs and systems of the body are affected and how severely affected they may be. In an attempt to classify these variations, a number of systems have been developed. The most commonly used is that formulated in 1979 by David Sillence, MD, which is descriptive. There are four main Sillence types, in which differences are based on clinical, radiographic, and genetic data (Table 1).

Type I, the most common, is the mildest form and is associated with blue sclerae (the usually white part of the eye), mild bone fragility, and normal teeth; decreased hearing is present in 50% of cases and there is minimal decrease in height.

Type II is the most severe form and is associated with blue sclerae, extreme bone fragility, cardiorespiratory failure, and extremely short stature; death often occurs before two years of age.

Type III is a severe form with wide variation in the degree of bone fragility and fracture rate, very short stature, blue or white sclerae, and dentinogenesis imperfecta (brittle teeth with abnormal dentin).

Type IV is moderate to severe in form with variation in the degree of bone fragility and fracture, short stature, white or gray sclerae, and dentinogenesis imperfecta.

Table 1. Characteristics of the Main Sillence Types of Osteogenesis Imperfecta.

Type	Severity	Genetics	Sclerae	Teeth	Bones	Scoliosis	Ambulatory Status (highly variable)
I	Mild	Autosomal dominant	Blue	Normal	Mild fragility	Rare	Independent in community
II	Frequently lethal	Autosomal dominant	Blue	?	Extreme fragility	Not applicable	Not applicable
III	Severe	Autosomal dominant or recessive (rare)	Blue or white	Dentino-genesis imperfecta	Moderate to severe fragility	Common	Some independent (without wheelchair) in community; most ambulatory in house with gait aids
IV	Moderate to severe	Autosomal dominant	Normal or gray	Dentino-genesis imperfecta	Moderate fragility	Common	Many independent (without wheelchair) in community

The mode of inheritance of all forms is autosomal dominant (not sex chromosome–linked and requiring only one copy of the abnormal dominant gene from either parent) with a rare case of recessive inheritance (requiring two copies of the abnormal recessive gene, one from each parent). In some children the genetic defect occurs as a spontaneous mutation with no family history of the disorder. Newer types (V, VI, and VII) have been added and are distinguished from the previous four by radiographic and histopathologic criteria. The Sillence system has been helpful in identifying general groups and has been very useful for stimulating research.

One shortcoming of this classification scheme is that it has little predictive capability for functional outcomes. It is limited in terms of identifying who is at greatest risk for disability and for which types of disability. Another classification system, formulated in 1993 by Helga Binder, MD, and colleagues, uses body size and the proportions of limbs, trunk, and head as well as measures of strength and motion as a way of predicting functional outcome. Function in this sense pertains to the ability to participate in life activities. The Binder scale seems to correlate well with independence in mobility and self-care.

Each type of osteogenesis imperfecta has a very wide variety of clinical features, or phenotypes. One of the most constant is bony abnormalities. These also vary widely. For example, some children have severe bowing of the long bones and others can have scoliosis, barrel chest, laxity of the joints, and joint deformities. All children with types II, III, and IV have short stature. All children with osteogenesis imperfecta are at increased risk for fracture, but this varies widely among and within the Sillence types. Not all affected children have fractures and many have them only infrequently. Fractured bone in osteogenesis imperfecta usually heals normally, but has to be properly aligned if it is to heal in the most advantageous position; some fractures develop bony overgrowth or excessive callus (in type V, for instance). Proper alignment can be achieved with splints, casts, or internal fixation using rods and pins, depending on the amount of bony displacement and the nature of the bone. External braces do not correct bowing, but can stabilize the bone by limiting motion. They substitute for weak muscles, thereby permitting relatively safe activity.

Most people with osteogenesis imperfecta have decreased muscle mass and strength, and the weakened muscles may not be capable of generating sufficient force to stress bone and stimulate it to grow. Bone development is dependent on muscle activity as well as on loading, or mechanical stress, through standing, walking, and lifting.

Children with osteogenesis imperfecta who are inactive or immobilized for specific treatments are at particular risk due to loss of muscle mass, given that they begin with less mass and cannot afford to lose any. Bone loses both structure and calcium from lack of motion and weight-bearing. In general, loss of muscle mass is quite rapid, reaching 10% per week if the muscle is fully immobilized. Recovery is likely to take longer than the immobilization period. For every week of immobilization, it is not uncommon to take two to three times longer to restore muscle strength. It can take as long as a year to restore muscle mass, even from one relatively short period of immobilization.

Some children with osteogenesis imperfecta have lax or hypermobile joints. This condition can contribute to instability at the joint and to less efficient use of muscle. Occasionally this laxity can involve the supporting structures of the skull, resulting in a settling of the skull on the upper part of the cervical spine and causing a condition known as basilar invagination. This condition can cause brain stem compression and neurological problems with abnormal reflexes and problems with muscle tone and strength. Research suggests this may progress slowly in many patients. It should be closely monitored. Surgery to stabilize the skull may be indicated to protect the brain stem and spine from injury.

The rehabilitation approach to evaluating and treating children with osteogenesis imperfecta starts with a thorough physical examination designed to determine the anatomical, mechanical, and developmental status of the child. A clinical "picture" is based on a composite of findings, including muscle strength, long bone bowing, joint alignment and laxity, chest proportions, pulmonary status, ratios and proportions of body segments, and patterns of limb movement. The child's temperament and comfort are also assessed. These findings are compared with observed performance of the child, and estimates are made about how these findings may limit function or delay development. Once this assessment is made, a treatment plan is put in place with goals designed to maximize the potential for function physically, psychologically, and socially.

The rehabilitation process, whether to restore or preserve function or to help manage recovery after surgery or fracture, should begin slowly. We recommend water activity as early as possible to encourage limb movement in all directions. Buoyancy helps limit stress on the limb, and pain, and keeps the amount of work the muscles have to do to a minimum. Bone that is osteoporotic can bend or fracture more readily than normal bone. Therapy should also include assistance for limb motion that supplements the effort of the recuperating child. The goal is to limit the forcefulness of muscular contraction so that the bone is relatively protected and to give the child a chance to move comfortably and independently. Water is the ideal medium for this.

Rehabilitative treatments often combine preventive and restorative techniques. For children with more significant weakness, especially trunk weakness, optimal seating is designed to maintain good trunk support to reduce stress from abnormal sitting postures that might contribute to scoliosis. Other treatment might include teaching parents and children how to solve mobility difficulties in a variety of environments. Most interventions attempt functional restoration and promote a healthy life style.

Many of the challenges faced by children with osteogenesis imperfecta can be addressed through a commitment to fitness and a healthy life style and the use of community and medical resources. The coordinated efforts of a multidisciplinary team of therapists, physicians, surgeons, nurses, teachers, family, and friends can assist children to reach a high level of performance, independence, and life satisfaction. The problems faced by children with osteogenesis imperfecta and their families are complex on several levels: anatomical, medical, adjustment to disability, and social. Some of these problems are formidable and may not be able to be completely solved; they may require adaptations and acceptance of limitations. If these challenges are to be managed in a fashion that promotes independence and good function, a thorough understanding of them is important.

Children with osteogenesis imperfecta rarely have difficulties with language or learning and are usually quite social and enthusiastic about school and family activities. In fact, with proper presentation they often welcome therapeutic intervention. The most common problems are weakness; abnormal body size, shape, and proportion; delays in mastery of gross motor targets; misalignment of long bones and joints; and pain. Occasionally there is associated pulmonary and cardiac dysfunction. In children with severe forms of the disease this can be the cause of death.

Clinical experience and published data suggest that body size and the ratio of head size to body length can influence performance and the achievement of developmental milestones, which can be delayed in osteogenesis imperfecta. Family members and others may notice that the child does not sit or hold the head up without support, or rolls over later than unaffected children. Identifying these delays begins an important process in terms of structuring the environment and devising interventional strategies to help infants master these activities. Successful treatments create opportunities for proper positioning and posture, for play activities that favor limb motion away from the body (such as reaching out and up), and for other movements that make muscles work against gravity (such as head lifting and the abdominal crunch).

Many early interventional strategies are designed to lay the groundwork for future more complex activities that depend on sufficient muscle strength and joint alignment. Identifying body asymmetries is crucial in designing corrective strategies. For example, correcting a leg length discrepancy using a proper lift can reduce stress on the lower back. Other examples include supporting the arch of the foot using a rigid orthotic device to enable more efficient gait and reduce stress on the knee joint; strengthening the muscle of the inner thigh to help realign the kneecap; and encouraging infants to turn to look to the side opposite a tight sternocleidomastoid muscle in the neck to help stretch the tight muscle responsible for torticollis, or wry neck. There is broad variation in the human developmental sequence. Not only do some children progress more slowly than others, but some do not pass through all of the "typical" stages. These variations are common among children and in those with osteogenesis imperfecta. However, when there is significant delay, treatment is required to accelerate mastery of critical developmental steps. Children with a large head out of proportion to trunk length and those with a barrel chest are at greatest risk for developmental delays. Sometimes these imbalances diminish as the child grows and sometimes they diminish in response to specific therapeutic interventions. The child's overall stature, or height, and muscle mass are predictors of function. Taller and stronger children can achieve a higher level of performance. Early appropriate treatment that addresses strength, alignment, and fitness can mitigate some of the anatomical disadvantages. Weight control, especially during late latency (an inactive period of bone growth) and early adolescence when weight gain is very high and often not accompanied by a significant growth spurt, increases the chance of achieving and sustaining ambulation and independent transfer from one position to another. As weight increases, the effort involved in walking and making transfers rises considerably, and the stress on weight-bearing long bones increases also. Increases in abdominal girth can strain the vertebral column, cause compression, and contribute to the development of such curvatures of the spine as scoliosis and kyphosis.

Generally speaking, children with osteogenesis imperfecta present the same range of variation as other children with regard to temperament. They also present the same range of variation as others with regard to their willingness to participate in therapy. When they reach adolescence, they often behave in a fashion similar to that of their nondisabled peers and resist doing what parents and others recommend. Routines that include exercise and sports activities are often accepted as a part of life if they can be introduced early, sustained through the latency years, and encouraged through adolescence.

Children who report pain do have pain. Their complaints should be respected and their pain should be controlled, especially since pain is usually underreported in children. Acute pain in the musculoskeletal system comes from bone or from soft tissue, such as muscle, tendon, or synovial membrane (the lining of joints). It can result from a muscle pull or a bruise or a bony fracture. The last can be a through-and-through break or a crack or microfracture that does not show up on x-ray film. Often you can tell the difference between them by the intensity and persistence of the crying or the child's lack of movement, which often accompanies an injured arm or leg. Back pain can result from compression fractures of the vertebrae, a nearly universal occurrence in children with osteogenesis imperfecta. Many of these compression fractures are silent. When children do not cry or verbalize pain but are in pain, their movement patterns are altered or they avoid moving the affected portion of the body. Chronic pain is sometimes more difficult to identify if the child cannot articulate its location or quality. Careful observation of the child's patterns of motion can give clues as to the presence and location of pain.

Children with severe forms of the disorder (type II and some with type III) can have cardiopulmonary involvement that can result in limitation of the delivery of oxygenated blood to the organs and muscles. Children with these findings have difficulty maintaining a reasonably high level of physical activity. They may need help in making transfers and may be unable to walk, and they can appear short of breath even with minimal or no physical effort. They occasionally have bluish lips. Viral and bacterial lung infections can cause severe breathing problems requiring antibiotics as well as supplemental oxygen. Nighttime oxygen may be required for acute episodes of infection and occasionally may be required continuously. Pulmonary function studies and sleep studies may be necessary to evaluate the children's status and medication may be required to treat problems of sleep apnea. These abnormalities can result from the collagen disorder itself or they can be a result of having severe scoliosis or some other chest deformity. There are no known exercises or postural strategies that can cure the cardiopulmonary problems. However, early emphasis on activities out of the wheelchair that focus on achieving upright position, attention to posture, proper chair fit, and good breathing techniques, can help with air exchange. Maintaining good muscle mass and strength can help promote efficiency of movement and delay the onset of chest muscle fatigue.

The chapters that follow build on the themes introduced here. They are organized by age group so that critical issues and treatments are discussed according to the events that should occur during infancy, childhood, and adolescence. Separate chapters explore adaptive equipment and devices likely to be beneficial, recommended sports and aquatics, and information resources we believe will be useful in networking with families and learning more about helping children with osteogenesis imperfecta.

CHAPTER TWO

STRATEGIES FOR INFANTS AND YOUNG CHILDREN

Early intervention to enhance performance and minimize impairment

Holly Lea Cintas, PT, PhD

Goals for infancy and early childhood, a period of dependence:

- To provide a wide variety of body positions to encourage environmental exploration and motor, perceptual, and cognitive development
- To achieve comfort and confidence as parents for holding, moving, playing with, and enjoying the baby with osteogenesis imperfecta
- To the extent possible, to provide the infant or child with the benefits of early prone experience to lay the groundwork for sitting, standing, and walking
- To identify and provide opportunities to build the child's sense of competence and independence

Introduction

Human infants require an extended period of protection and nurturing before achieving effective locomotion and the ability to feed themselves. Thus, it is reasonable that infants with osteogenesis imperfecta require caregiver support for some time before they gain independence in mobility and feeding. On the other hand, babies and young children without motor limitations often complete all major locomotor transitions in their first year of life, beginning with rolling, then progressing to sitting, standing, and walking. Parents of infants with osteogenesis imperfecta face a unique dilemma: how much to challenge their babies to encourage motor performance and reinforce a positive association with it, while at the same time minimizing the risk for fracture and for reinforcing dependency and failure.

Infancy is a window of opportunity for children with osteogenesis imperfecta. This chapter describes strategies to encourage exploration, and the gradual achievement of independence, while at the same time building the child's concept of competence or "can do." The early intervention concepts described in this chapter take into account the fact that infants and children with osteogenesis imperfecta have widely varying temperaments, and physical capabilities. Thus, the concepts are general, described according to performance level and target objective. They are not directed to specific types of osteogenesis imperfecta because of the wide performance variation within each type. While the activities described below are applicable for babies with a wide range of capability, an individualized program, tailored to a specific child's needs, is always preferable to the application of general concepts.

First Things First

Infants have developed all the motor patterns they will have at birth as a 20-week fetus, but they appear relatively immobile as neonates because of confinement with growth, and long periods of sleep during the last 4 months of gestation. Thus, it takes time for the infant to recover from the confinement, adapt to the new space available, and learn to function in an environment that requires antigravity competence.

Neonatal motor capabilities vary widely, depending on cultural heritage, temperament, and body type, but generally the kinetic behavior of infants is linked to their temperament. Some babies are low-key and placid, easily satisfied, and move relatively little. Others are fussy or highly kinetic or both, although most infants display a blend of these qualities. It is crucial to remember that infants with osteogenesis imperfecta are individuals. Achieving our goals will depend on the ability to synchronize our efforts with the child's temperament and capabilities.

Intervention strategies for the youngest infants include the use of:
- Different body positions to provide opportunities for the infant to learn to move muscles and joints against gravity

- An aquatic medium to encourage the infant's independent efforts and a growing sense of competence
- Parent carrying positions to modify body alignment (especially the legs) and to encourage the development of head control

Body Positions and Related Activities

Backlying, or supine, is the most common position for caregiving. It provides opportunity for sustained social contact, and since the body is fully supported by the support surface, the reclining infant is usually comfortable, risk-free, and relatively unchallenged from the standpoint of antigravity motor skill. Usually it is not necessary for a baby with osteogenesis imperfecta to be placed on egg crate material or on an air mattress, which actually makes it more difficult for the baby to initiate and control movements. Diapering is done in supine by lifting the infant's bottom while supporting both legs at the same time in order to place the diaper under the pelvis. It is crucial to train all caregivers to avoid lifting the baby's body by pulling on one or both legs.

In the hospital during the neonatal period, the baby can be gently eased from the back toward *sidelying* using a towel roll or sandbag behind the baby's back. At first the goal should be only a few degrees, then a quarter turn, then a half turn (45 degrees), gradually accomplishing a comfortable and secure sidelying position in each direction. It can be helpful to place a towel or washcloth roll in front of the infant, well below the face, to be certain the baby doesn't roll forward abruptly. Progression toward *prone* position (lying on the tummy) should be done from sidelying toward prone in the same manner as described above, only a few degrees at time, so that the infant can adapt comfortably to the gradual progression. Additional strategies to accomplish prone position in a conservative manner are described below.

Once the baby is at home, after each diaper change during the day, it's easy to remember to do a little work on neck strengthening. With the baby backlying, begin by lifting both the baby's shoulders, placing your arms behind the shoulders, very gently off the support surface less than an inch, four or five times, so the neck muscles gradually start taking responsibility for holding the head. The shoulders should not be lifted so high that the head is unsupported. If the baby becomes unhappy or starts to resist, the challenge is too much. Either don't lift the shoulders quite as high or reduce the number of repetitions until the baby is comfortable with the routine again. The eventual goal is for the infant to have complete control of the head for the trip up into sitting. This generally takes several months to accomplish.

Kicking is a skill the infant can practice when positioned in supine, but often young infants with osteogenesis imperfecta have difficulty doing this because of weakness. In backlying, the legs often remain open and widely spaced on the support surface, an appropriate position for a neonate, but one from which an infant should transition fairly quickly. For infants with osteogenesis imperfecta, elevation of the legs off the support surface and the achievement of kicking are hastened by experience in water, infor-

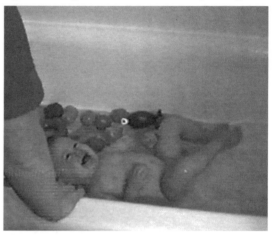

Figure 1. Using the buoyancy of water to bring the legs up and together for kicking.

mally called the *waterworks* program. Placing the infant flat on the back on the bottom of a conventional bathtub (padded with a thick towel or foam) in 2 to 3 inches of warm water, no clothing, often provides just enough buoyancy to help the baby bring the legs up and together to kick (Figure 1). It's all right if water gets in the ears; it was there throughout the gestational period. However, if this is a concern or the baby gets ear infections easily, the head can be elevated with a soft support. The key is that the baby should be comfortable and happy. Just talking and smiling at young infants usually is enough to get them to start kicking. Often one has the feeling that they can't resist your charms and simply have to kick as part of their general excitement.

Kicking in water can begin while the baby is in the hospital, using a blanket to fully support the baby's body, legs, and arms during the trip into and out of a plastic bassinet with approximately 2 to 3 inches of warm water. However, starting at home is appropriate for most families. Waterworks should be done for about 20 to 30 minutes once a day; it's even better if it can be done twice a day. It often works best as simply a play time, not associated with the infant's bath, because the two together may be too tiring. If the baby does not like this activity, don't persist, but starting with the baby dressed in the water may help solve the problem. It is useful to continue kicking in water as a specific intervention until the baby can kick on dry land, lifting each leg completely up and off the support surface toward midline, one leg at a time or both legs coming up together. This usually takes between 2 weeks and 3 months to achieve.

Kicking in water should be an entirely positive experience designed to:
- Build a satisfying association with movement for the baby
- Provide the infant with very early experience in moving entirely by one-self, unaided by someone else, thus beginning the groundwork for developing self-competence
- Accelerate a skill that could take much longer to accomplish out of the water
- Provide parents and babies with mutually satisfying opportunities for play

Reaching can be encouraged in the supine position both in and out of water, but it is usually easier to begin reaching while sidelying because it is more difficult to reach upward against gravity while backlying on land or in water. Infants usually respond best by reaching for a very colorful (including black and white) object at fairly close range, which doesn't require significant effort. If too much effort is required, the infant will learn to give up quickly. This principle also holds for older children, and even for adults, when it comes to exercise, and it reinforces failure rather than success. The key is to keep it fun, and the individual will often want to continue the activity and gradually increase the amount of effort.

A second very important principle for infants is to give them the object they reach for, each time, if they have successfully contacted it. Failing to do so will extinguish the behavior rapidly. If you want the infant to reach again, present a different object, and let the baby explore the significance of having one in each hand or placing it in the mouth. When the infant is losing interest, present still another object to maintain the novelty of the situation, positioned in a manner that elicits the motor behavior you want while providing an interesting experience for the baby. This process is intended to be playful, can rarely be sustained beyond a few minutes, and should be discontinued when the baby, or the caregiver, loses interest.

Body positions other than backlying provide interactive opportunities for the baby's body and brain to learn from the environment. A further advantage is to minimize the tendency for the infant's head to become flattened on the back. This happens occasionally when infants are ill or immobilized for prolonged periods and have had to spend most of their time in backlying position. In most cases, this is easily remediated by alternating body positions among backlying, sidelying with gradual progression toward lying on the tummy, and supported sitting in a reclined position. For children who do not have osteogenesis imperfecta, use of a helmet or band to mold the head sometimes is considered if an infant has significant right-left asymmetry of the skull. However, this is rarely indicated for flattening of the back of the head, particularly for children with osteogenesis imperfecta, since the additional weight of the helmet makes it very difficult for the baby to move the head or the body.

Infants with osteogenesis imperfecta may have ***torticollis***, an asymmetry of the neck in which the head is tilted toward one side and the face is usually rotated to the opposite side. The baby's head appears closer to one shoulder than the other. Many factors contribute to this asymmetry, including the baby's body position during pregnancy and muscle weakness. An x-ray or MRI of the neck may be necessary to rule out nonmuscular factors as the source of the asymmetry.

Exercise interventions for torticollis are specific for an individual child, but generally focus on active exercise of the muscles that pull the head in the opposite direction. For example, lifting the baby upward from a position of right sidelying elicits muscle action on the left side of the neck if the baby's head, although carefully supported, is held slightly lower than the body while coming up. Passive stretching is rarely successful because the infant learns to fight it almost immediately. Please refer to the discussion of torticollis and general principles for intervention in the section below on building a better back and trunk.

Sidelying is useful, as noted above, to begin reaching activities but it also provides several additional benefits. It brings the legs closer together to prepare for sitting and standing, it helps to position the head in the middle, and it gives the baby the benefit of working the arms, legs, head, and trunk (torso) against gravity in a completely different orientation than when on the back or tummy. Although positioning seems passive with respect to infant care, varied positions provide infants opportunities to develop competence in all planes of movement. In general, for young infants who do not roll or have locomotor capability, it is an advantage to change their body position every 20 to 30 minutes while they are awake. It is not necessary to change the baby's position during sleep.

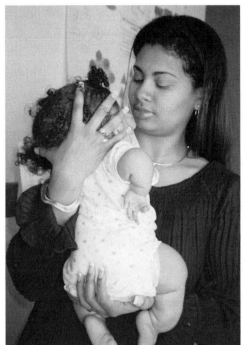

Lying in *prone position* (on the tummy) is a challenging skill for all infants. This is especially the case for infants with osteogenesis imperfecta because of caregivers' concern about rib fractures, larger than average head size, and weakness of the muscles that extend the back and neck to lift the head. When positioned in prone, infants have to be able to lift the head enough to clear the face to breathe. They will be frantic if placed in that position when they can't. If infants are forced to do this before they are ready, a bad association with this position may begin, progressing to the infant's refusal to accommodate to this position at all. Fortunately, this can be avoided or resolved fairly easily with a slow progression within the infant's tolerance.

Figure 2. Achieving upright head control while facing the caregiver's shoulder.

Infants with osteogenesis imperfecta can accomplish tummy lying and head elevation through a series of gradual steps designed to achieve this essential competency. The easiest way is to start upright, with the baby facing the parent's shoulder (Figure 2). Support the head in back, of course, but give the infant a chance to take responsibility for holding the head a bit while positioned slightly away from the shoulder. This should be done for brief periods, always stopping before the baby becomes fatigued or fretful. It is important to alternate right and left shoulders so the infant has experience on both sides of the parent's body. Some parents organize this so that one parent always carries the infant against the right shoulder, the other against the left.

When this skill is coming along nicely, the next step is to position the baby face-to-face on the parent's or caregiver's chest (Figure 3). The parent sits on a sofa or in a soft chair for a few minutes two or three times a day, gradually reclining over a period of days

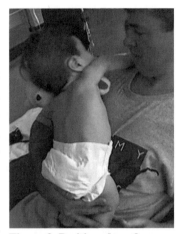

Figure 3. Positioned on the parent's chest to encourage head elevation and reaching in prone.

or weeks, so the baby adjusts to going lower and lower in a comfortable position adjacent to the parent. The objective is to encourage the baby to try to lift the head during this progression. Sometimes this occurs when the reclining parent talks to the baby. Sometimes it requires the other parent or a caregiver positioned behind or to the side of the

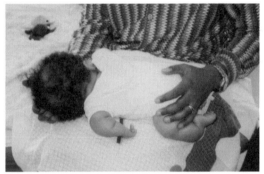

Figure 4. In prone, positioned on Dad's knees; note that the child's forehead is supported by her father's hand.

baby with an interesting toy or comment to encourage head lifting and turning. Once again, it is crucial to stop and change to another activity while the baby is still succeeding, rather than push to the point of fatigue or failure.

The next step is the transition to a different support surface. This can be to the parent's knees (Figure 4), briefly, and then to a firmer base, such as the floor, with a soft carpet or, in the absence of carpeting, a mat or thick towel to ensure protection of the face if the baby's head bobs. A crib mattress is a good surface, but only with complete supervision. It is much easier for the infant to

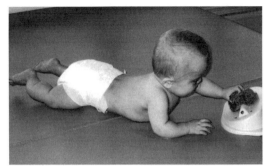

Figure 5. Head elevation as a preliminary to shifting the body to one side in order to reach.

stabilize the body to lift the head on a firm surface. A soft, pliant surface such as an adult's bed, a piece of foam, or a very thick blanket makes this task much harder and is unsafe.

Once the baby can lift and turn the head to clear the face comfortably, the next step is to encourage lifting the head up a bit higher with the forearms tucked under the chest to begin forearm weight-bearing. This skill offers even more head elevation, a prerequisite for the skills listed below.

Head elevation in prone position is the gateway to:
- Rolling over from tummy to back
- Shifting bodyweight onto one side in order to reach with the opposite arm (Figure 5)
- Rotating the body in a circle or pushing backward while on the tummy
- Pulling forward while on the tummy and eventually pushing up off the floor

Building a Better Back and Trunk

Babies may be more socially engaging when lying supine, but we emphasized above the importance of providing prone experience to strengthen the back and neck muscles in anticipation of sitting and standing. While the effect of weakness of the arms or legs is obvious (the baby can't reach overhead or lift the legs to kick), the crucial role of the trunk (the back and *front* of the mid-portion of the body), in supporting independent movement is less apparent, but extremely important. The arms and legs literally hang from the trunk and their muscles must stabilize on the trunk in order to move. Thus, it is as important to strengthen the trunk as the arms and legs in order to increase movement capability. As described above, this occurs during backlying for muscles on the front of the neck, chest, and abdomen through activities such as reaching, lifting the legs to kick, and transitions from supine to sitting, which begin with gently lifting the baby's shoulders, caregiver's hands behind the shoulders, in supine to elicit anterior neck control. Notably, the neck and abdominal muscles work together to accomplish lifting the head. The same thing is true for the muscles on the back of the neck and the back of the trunk. The head can move independently of the trunk by means of the joints in the neck, but like the arms and legs, it gains stability through muscular insertions on the trunk. For example, an infant lifting the head while lying on the tummy appears to be simply elevating the head, but achieving this requires stabilization of the joints all the way down the spine. And this is achieved through *opportunity* (being placed in the prone or preprone positions described above) and *practice* (learning how to elevate the head in space in different body positions).

Infants and young children with osteogenesis imperfecta occasionally have **torticollis**, in which the head tilts to one side, and most often, rotates to the opposite side. This can result from several factors, including, as noted above, the baby's position during pregnancy and neck muscle weakness. Rarely, a problem exists in the bony segments of the neck, especially when the head is tilted and also rotated to the same side. An x-ray or an MRI (magnetic resonance imaging) of the neck may be necessary to rule out vertebral malalignment or other contributing factors before beginning an intervention program to improve head and neck alignment.

Passive stretching is generally unsuccessful even in very young infants because they learn to fight it almost immediately, and this becomes a battleground for parents and child. Active neck movements, elicited by the caregiver, are safer and more effective for children with torticollis and osteogenesis imperfecta.

Interventions for torticollis are specific for individual children, but several general concepts are relevant (examples described for one side also apply to the opposite side):
- If the head is tilted to the right, placing the infant in right sidelying for significantly more time than left sidelying encourages head orientation toward midline. Encouraging rolling from backlying to right sidelying also encourages midline alignment.
- If the head is tilted to the right, lifting the baby from right sidelying, with

the head well supported but held slightly below the body, selectively activates the muscles on the left side of the neck to pull the head toward midline.

• Placing the infant on a relatively firm surface in prone with a toy positioned on the left side within easy reach encourages the baby to rotate the head to the left side. The task must be easy and successfully completed in order to get the baby to do it again (using a different toy).

• If the child is lacking head turning to the left, placing the baby with the head turned toward the left gently and momentarily in prone after each diaper change over the course of a day adds up and can be surprisingly effective. Pick the baby up immediately if he or she complains. This can be attempted three or four times quickly after each diaper change so it becomes a game.

• Observing the baby's head while being carried (facing the parent) reveals whether the parent's right or left shoulder is the best place to encourage the baby to rotate the head in the preferred direction. It may be wise to carry the baby that way until head turning equalizes, then go back to alternating shoulders. A similar analysis should be used to determine which elbow is best (in the baby's face-forward carrying position) to promote midline head position for an infant with torticollis.

• These activities are effective if carried out briefly several times during the day. They should be done in a manner that is slightly challenging but not uncomfortable for the infant because the goal is to develop a positive association with physical effort.

Long-term objectives for the neck, back, and trunk include:
• Sufficient strength to permit the head, neck, arms, and legs to function against gravity
• Best spinal alignment that can be achieved, including the head in midline and the longest, straightest back
• Early use of positions and related activities for younger infants and children to lay the groundwork for optimal function and alignment later

Transitions: From Body Positions to Encouraging Active Movement

Rolling begins with using the static positions described above to start the process of moving between them. Although many techniques to encourage rolling are done with hands-on manipulation by a caregiver, this probably should be avoided for children with osteogenesis imperfecta, since imposed rotation is risky. Rather, active rolling can be encouraged safely for infants with osteogenesis imperfecta, and this approach offers the bonus of building in the child's discovery of independent achievement.

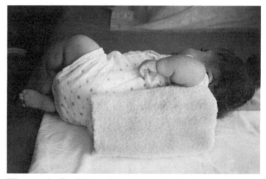

Positioning in sidelying offers a good example of positioning to limit movement versus positioning to encourage movement. Placing a towel roll or other positioning device in front of and behind the sidelying infant ensures, to

Figure 6. Positioned in sidelying (using a towel roll) as a preliminary to rolling forward or backward; the child's legs are fully supported on the table.

a large extent, that the infant will stay in that position, but it also limits the child's independent efforts. We suggest that, after the neonatal period, once the child is comfortable in sidelying, using a towel roll only in the front or the back will provide some sidelying experience and will not limit the baby's efforts to explore the available space (Figure 6). Placing the roll behind the baby, with some interesting objects in front within sight and reaching range, encourages active reaching toward the object, linked with rolling toward prone (on the abdomen).

Progression from sidelying to prone can also be facilitated by placing the towel roll in front of the infant and positioning the baby toward prone at various points in a sequence along the 90 degree arc between sidelying and prone, so the transition is very gradual and easily accepted. Consider these positioning strategies as part of the intervention program, rather than positioning to walk away, because they will not be tolerated for more than 5 to 10 minutes at a time initially.

Rolling from sidelying to backlying can be achieved in the same manner. If infants are not "locked in" with positioning devices, they will usually discover how to do this independently. This can also be encouraged by placing the infant slightly behind sidelying (about 15 degrees toward supine), towel roll or other support behind the back, then presenting an object of interest from behind the baby's head and upper shoulder, so the baby looks backward and rolls slightly back to reach it.

Recalling the discussion above on the linkages between the trunk and extremities (arms and legs), the reach described above is the obvious motor behavior. However, while reaching forward, the infant activates muscles on the front of the trunk that pull the head forward and flex the trunk in the middle, thus practicing the very patterns needed to roll from back to tummy, and later, to sit up. Similarly, reaching backward while in sidelying activates muscles on the back of the neck and trunk that lift the head, extend the back, and support the roll from tummy to back, and later, locomotion in prone.

Sitting presents the challenge of balancing the development of good back and trunk alignment while at the same time encouraging independent behavior. Use of supportive infant seats is common in North America. For short periods, they benefit the parents, bring the infant into the social scene, and provide an alternative to backlying. However, it is advantageous to change an awake baby's position to sidelying or prone after sitting passively for 30 minutes in a flexed forward posture. This may not always be possible, especially in the car, but avoiding many hours of sitting in a flexed-forward position can be useful over the long term for improved back alignment.

In a similar manner, awareness of right-left body symmetry is important for the young infant or child sitting passively. An occasional head tilt to one side for short periods, in a car seat, for example, is of little concern. A chronic tendency to tilt the head to the same side is important and should be addressed early, as discussed above for torticollis. For the infant without anti-gravity head control, the head can be positioned in midline in a car seat or infant seat with a boppy cushion (see Chapter 7 for a description), or a washcloth or other soft roll with attention to not locking the child's head in place or obscuring the visual field. Alternating parents' carrying positions between the baby facing their right or left shoulders is also an important consideration for encouraging head in midline as preparation for sitting. For the child with antigravity head control, asymmetry of the neck or trunk is addressed through specific active exercises for that child to balance the muscular forces on the neck, as well as positioning to encourage better alignment, as discussed above for torticollis. Careful consideration of the sitting devices the child is using is important to ensure the best possible alignment, and that the devices themselves are not contributing to the asymmetry.

The transition from passive, supported sitting to *active sitting* begins when the infant has sufficient head control to maintain the head comfortably upright and in midline for short periods. Often the baby demonstrates this by trying to pull forward out of the infant seat, or push backward from the caregiver's shoulder when being carried upright. Preliminaries to active sitting include those described above: learning to take responsibility for holding the head on the trip up from supine to sitting, and learning to lift the head, and rotate it to look around, when lying in prone on the parent's chest, or knees, or on the floor on a blanket.

It seems obvious that an aggressive approach to achieving active sitting when the child doesn't have head control is not a good idea, if long-term back alignment is important. Thus, short bursts of active sitting during the day are preferred, rather than striving to increase the length of time in sitting, especially if back and head alignment are not optimal. It is often easiest to start this with the caregiver

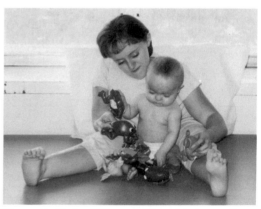

Figure 7. Early sitting; positioned between the caregiver's open legs, the child can alternate reaching down toward the floor with reaching up and above the head for toys.

sitting on the floor, baby positioned in sitting facing forward, legs extended, between the parent's open, extended legs (Figure 7). This position provides good support for the pelvis so the child can weave and bob a little but still sit securely against the parent's inner thighs. Initially, this should be done for very short periods, 1 to 5 minutes, until the infant builds up tolerance and it remains an interesting thing to do rather than something to endure.

Toys can be put on the floor in front of the child, but even at this early stage, it is advantageous to bias the back toward extension, or an erect position. Presenting the toys from behind the child or placing them on a box, stool, or tray at the level of the child's chest promotes a more erect posture. For the same reason, even though propped sitting (supporting oneself by leaning forward and resting on the hands) is viewed by some as a milestone on the road to independence, it is not recommended for infants and children with osteogenesis imperfecta. It encourages sustained trunk flexion (forward bending in sitting) and excessive hip flexion, positions the child will spend many years trying to minimize. Also, if the child falls forward abruptly from propped sitting, there is risk of a femoral fracture. It is much easier to build a straighter, more erect back than to try to extend it later. Once the child has achieved good back extension in sitting, it is very easy to learn to reach down forward or sideways to pick up toys on the floor.

Sitting semisupported on the floor can be complemented by a parent carrying position in which the child faces forward, pelvis tucked into one arm of the caregiver, legs together over the parent's supporting arm. This gives the child some responsibility for maintaining sitting while at the same time encouraging legs together in preparation for standing and walking.

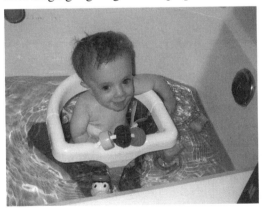

Figure 8. Sitting in the bathtub.

Sitting in the bathtub can begin when the child can sit (outside the tub) with an erect, symmetrical back and minimal external support, for example, with a pillow or a parent behind the sitting child. *Constant supervision by a parent or other caregiver is essential* whether the child sits in the tub in a ring suction-cupped to the bottom (Figure 8) or with no support device. In either case, this is a great opportunity for reaching, batting, or just playing in the water. All of these activities contribute to weight-shifting practice in sitting with the protective advantage of the support of the water around the trunk (the pelvis and chest).

When the child is comfortable sitting on the floor (not in water) with legs straight in front (long sitting) or flexed and crossed (tailor or ring sitting), *interventions to improve sitting out of water diverge in two different directions:*

- Transitions from sitting still on the floor (static sitting) to weight-shifting while sitting in order to progress to moving in and out of sitting and scooting
- Sitting on a higher surface (a parent's thigh, small stool, or large book) with hips and knees flexed and feet flat on the floor (short sitting or 90/90/90 degree position) to increase the challenge of maintaining an upright position and to begin weight-bearing on the feet

Transitions into and out of sitting are often manually facilitated by physical therapists through active hands-on weight-shifting, sometimes using a therapy ball. Imposing movement on children with osteogenesis imperfecta, particularly on an unstable surface, creates an element of risk that may be undesirable. The same motor behaviors can be elicited by structuring the environment so the child can perform actively, and securely, within safe boundaries that only the child feels. For example, for a child sitting on the floor, placing toys or other desirable objects in locations that require a reach and a minimal body weight shift is a good starting point. It is critical that this be a minimal effort to begin, rather than so scary that the child won't do it again. Objects can be placed on the floor in front, to the side, and perhaps very slightly to the back of the child to encourage reaching for them. More importantly, desirable objects can be presented all the way from the base point (the floor) to the top of the child's ability to reach overhead securely and without fear of falling. For children with osteogenesis imperfecta, it is less important to reach across midline than to practice different trajectories that encourage weight-shifting of the body axis forward, to the side, and backward (reaching above the head). Once again, when the child grasps the toy, it should not be taken away to repeat the task. Another toy should be presented after allowing for a period of exploration of the toy or desirable object just obtained.

Another approach to achieving weight-shifting of the body's central axis or trunk into or out of sitting is to put a high, soft pillow to the side and have the child lie down on it and get up again, with a little manual assistance if needed. The same thing can be done by positioning the pillow halfway between the child's side and the back, and then behind the back, so the child practices getting up and getting down in a circle of positions all around the body except in front. It is preferable to minimize down and up transitions with the pillow in front because the objective is to limit activities that promote a rounded back, with the obvious exception of an occasional reach downward for a toy. In addition, it is wise to avoid encouraging a transition from sitting to pronelying by having the child roll forward onto the abdomen through widely open legs. This is risky in terms of the potential for femoral fracture and can be done instead by having the child "lie down" from sitting onto a high, soft pillow, then roll over onto the tummy and scoot down backward off the pillow. With increasing skill and confidence, lower and lower pillows or other soft surfaces can be used until the child can rotate the body and move out of sitting with no external support.

The same methods can be used to transition from backlying or pronelying upward into sitting if the child is encouraged to roll sideways onto a low pillow and given some instruction to push up with the arms while in sidelying, receiving a little external assistance from a caregiver to support the trunk and the pelvis on the way up. Getting up requires much more care than getting down to avoid too much stress on the arms, so the child's responsibility for arm support should be increased very gradually. Generally, even young children will know, and will show you how much they can safely push up without getting into trouble.

Efforts directed to accomplish scooting in sitting can begin at the same time as transitions into and out of sitting by learning to scoot in a circle on the floor, a tiny bit at a time to begin. Strategies to achieve this are described below under locomotion.

Active sitting above the floor (short sitting) in preparation for standing begins when the child can sit erect with the head in midline rather than falling to one side, and the back is relatively straight rather than drooping forward or sideways. This activity can occur in many ways. A good place to begin is to place the child in sitting on the caregiver's thigh, knees together, facing outward, or same position, child sitting on one thigh and facing inward toward the caregiver's opposite thigh (Figure 9A). This is an important variation from the way this activity is often done for infants and children just learning to sit and stand, whose legs are positioned open, over the caregiver's thigh, facing the foot. While this open legs position may be appropriate for other children who need to develop a wide base of support, infants and children with osteogenesis imperfecta typically have widely spaced, outwardly rotated legs. Thus, it is preferable to position the thighs as close together as is comfortable; the feet can be up to 1 to 2 inches apart, but flat on the floor.

Sitting this way with minimal or no back support (the caregiver's hands are usually at the pelvis) begins for only a few minutes at a time, and lasts only as long as the child is comfortable and sitting posture is good. Activities in this position can include simply sitting and talking (Figure 9B) or singing, since the child is already challenged

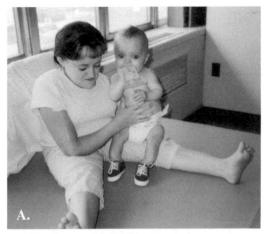

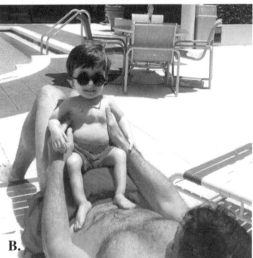

Figure 9. Two approaches to early weight-bearing; the children's knees could be a bit closer together.

to sit erect without back support and is weight-bearing on the feet during this static sitting. Progressions include reaching or throwing in this position to encourage comfortable and secure weight-shifting; for example, giving the child a ball to throw to another caregiver who can retrieve it and give it back to the child to throw again. These activities not only encourage weight-shifting of the trunk in sitting, but are also the basis for early, safe weight-bearing experiences for the child's feet.

Transitions to other sitting positions include placing the seated child on a low stool or other very firm surface facing the caregiver, knees together and feet on the floor, supporting the child at the pelvis so a fall cannot occur. With increased tolerance, the child can sit in a highchair at the table or upright in a stroller, with knees together and foot support in both cases. Comfortable foam pads placed in the highchair or stroller can be used to encourage a position of legs together rather than widely spaced. Carrying the child facing forward with pelvis tucked into the elbow and legs flexed forward over the parent's flexed forearm will also reinforce short sitting and legs together. Based on the discussion above, it should be obvious that the child has to have good head and trunk control before being placed in these positions for several minutes.

Active standing is easiest to begin on the floor, the child sitting on the caregiver's thigh with the child's legs fairly close together, feet 1 to 2 inches apart. This is a very low challenge for weight-bearing on the feet, which can be increased gradually through reaching forward and to the side for desirable objects, gradually shifting weight over the feet. When the child is comfortable sitting and moving in this position, the next step is to gently lift the child at the pelvis as if the child were going to stand up, but only go up about an inch and then sit down again. If this is done conservatively, it shouldn't be scary and can be repeated three or four times.

If the child responds poorly, don't try it again until the next day, and then do it only once. A very gradual ascent in this skill, as in any other, is built on a succession of increasing successes, rather than on pushing so hard that everyone involved fails. In most cases, the child begins to take over the responsibility for standing up, so the caregiver does less and less. The goal is to make it fun so that the child, hopefully, looks forward to standing and enjoys doing it, with external support, of course.

Shortly after beginning active standing, it is important to look at the position of the child's loaded feet while barefoot. If they are completely flat, it might be wise to consider using a plantar contact (bottom of the foot only) orthotic device in a sneaker to support the arches on the inside of the foot during imposed standing. On the one hand, infants and children without osteogenesis imperfecta often do not have arches when they begin standing, but they are in control of the progression to achieve standing and walking. On the other hand, high-performing children and adolescents with osteogenesis imperfecta often have completely flat feet that limit their function. Their standing progression has typically been imposed by caregivers, rather than initiated by the young child.

It seems logical for the child to practice standing with the body segments in the best alignment. Since the hyperflexibility associated with osteogenesis imperfecta is especially prevalent in the weight-bearing joints of the feet, why not support them during early, imposed weight-bearing? If the heel bone (calcaneus) is right under the Achilles tendon (in the middle of the back of the calf) during standing and the medial arch is low, an off-the-shelf plantar contact orthotic device is sufficient to elevate the arch and improve stability in standing. If the heel bones are significantly swayed outward or inward during standing, the child may need an orthosis that comes above the heel. The rehabilitation physician, orthopedist, and physical therapist can help determine which type of orthotic device or orthosis is the best choice for a specific child.

Sit-to-stand from the caregiver's thigh or a stool, with external pelvic support, gradually transitions to using the sofa or a similar piece of furniture to pull up to standing, allowing children to take as much responsibility for doing this as they wish. Although the feet may be several inches apart, they should be positioned straight ahead for this activity at the starting position. To minimize the risk of fracture, the feet or legs should not be rotated by the caregiver once the child starts to put weight on them. Once again the key is to have fun with this and to link it to playing with toys on the support surface (a sofa or shelf), talking, singing, or reaching, for example. It is much more effective to have children sit down or get down before they are fatigued, and stand again later, than to prolong the period of standing until it becomes uncomfortable or unpleasant, thereby decreasing interest in repeating this.

From standing at the couch or sofa, the transition is turning sideways to walk forward (with manual support or a walker) for children with osteogenesis imperfecta rather than encouraging sidestepping or cruising, which promotes a legs-open position and a wide base of support. Of course, the child can independently sidestep to move from one piece of furniture to another in the course of development, and shouldn't be prevented from doing this. However, one consideration is to simply avoid practicing sidestepping as a therapeutic activity, since minimizing the legs-wide-open position is a constant challenge related to sitting, standing, and walking.

Active standing for short periods can be complemented by *passive standing* using adaptive devices. For children older than 2 years who have never stood or walked, long leg braces with a pelvic band, called an HKAFO (hip, knee, ankle, foot orthosis), occasionally are used to provide the ability to stand instantly when the knee and hip joints on the braces are locked. Used in this manner, the braces provide an external source of stability, but are not a means of reducing the incidence of fractures. Long leg bracing is a very expensive approach, as well as labor-intensive in terms of putting on and taking off the braces, worn only for standing and walking. However, it provides the stability to go from standing to walking very quickly in the parallel bars, followed by transition to a walker or crutches. This approach is particularly useful for children with significant hip muscle weakness, and can provide a sense of security for some children and parents. Once the child has gained the skill, the knee joints are gradually unlocked, and the child is eased out of using the braces for standing and walking as the muscles become stronger as a result of exercises and especially active standing strategies. In other words, the opportunity to stand and walk in the braces promotes this skill, but is rarely sufficient to gain the strength to walk without them unless strengthening exercises are occurring at the same time, that is, active standing, and arm, trunk, and leg exercises. Many types of passive standing devices other than braces are available (also see Chapter 7).

Three general categories of standing devices are:
- *Supine standers,* on which the child lies down on the back and is brought up to standing gradually
- *Prone standers,* which are already somewhat upright when the child is placed on the device in prone position (on the abdomen)
- *Upright standers,* which are completely upright and the child takes full weight-bearing on the feet when placed on the stander

For most children with osteogenesis imperfecta, supine standers work best because they can be elevated gradually, shifting the body weight from the back to the feet at a rate that is comfortable for the child. Another advantage is that the child can easily be taken off the supine stander while lying down if there is a problem. This is not the case with prone or upright standers on which the child is immediately weight-bearing on the feet when placed in the stander or has to lie flat on the abdomen to begin. Prone standers are highly appropriate for children with low muscle tone associated with neurological dysfunction to bring up their trunk and extremity tone. But they are not usually recommended for children with osteogenesis imperfecta because of the difficulty of achieving a gradual ascent. Upright standers, some of which can be self-propelled, are useful for older children with osteogenesis imperfecta who can already stand comfortably. This introduces the issue of how long the child should stay in the stander.

Very young children with osteogenesis imperfecta generally do not adapt to standers well because they are often quite mobile and won't tolerate being strapped into a passive standing device. Occasionally they will adjust if the length of time in the device is brought up very slowly, but generally they do much better with the active standing strategies described above or long leg braces. It is particularly important to avoid forcing a young child to stay in the stander because it builds a negative association with standing, an undesirable outcome if the objective is to encourage that behavior.

Older children (see Chapters 3 and 4) generally tolerate supine standers well for 30 to 45 minutes once or twice a day, particularly if they have already been standing or walking. These are useful to maintain standing during recovery from a fractured arm when the child cannot use crutches or a walker, or as a gradual way to reintroduce weight-bearing on the legs after surgery or a fracture. The angle of the stander and the amount of time in the device are determined according to the comfort, perception of safety, and tolerance of the child. Frequently when children reach middle school, they refuse to use a stander at school because of concerns about how they appear to their classmates. In those instances, parents may wish to use devices at home to maintain or reestablish standing.

Locomotion

The concepts and strategies discussed above are preparatory to the ability to move in space. The goal of this section is to consider all possible types of locomotion for a young child with osteogenesis imperfecta and how to encourage development of a variety of them. Strange as it may seem, clothing restraint is the place to begin. To the same extent that parents come home from work and change into something more comfortable, infants and children need to be able to move comfortably without being restrained by clothing. This means avoiding clothing with tight necks and tight shoulders, tight socks and pant legs, and dresses for infants and young girls learning to crawl or pull up to standing. Jeans are cute on very young children, but are heavy and often constraining for an active infant or child. Slippery shorts or pants can be helpful to facilitate movement for older children, but may be a bit risky for young ones, depending on the child, the body proportions, and the floor surface. The key is an awareness of clothing choices that make movement as easy as possible for the child, and encourage the child's earliest efforts to help with undressing and dressing.

Scooting on the back by pushing with the feet may be the child's first type of locomotion. This is an important life skill; everyone should be able to do it, including infants and children with osteogenesis imperfecta. Older children often use this strategy to move after coming out of a spica cast. However, to the extent possible, every effort should be made to ensure that this is not the child's only means of locomotion. In addition to the toll it takes on the hair on the back of the head, scooting on the back does not link to antigravity behaviors or support progress to higher developmental skills. Rolling, in contrast, presents an antigravity challenge for the neck, arms, legs, and trunk, and lays the groundwork for more complex locomotor behaviors.

Sequential rolling is more likely to be an infant's or child's first type of locomotion. Simply a matter of stringing together a series of rolls in one direction, rolling has multiple benefits for children with osteogenesis imperfecta at all ages. It promotes an extended body position and activates muscle groups over the entire length of the body. Rolling requires coordinated movement of the neck, back, arms, and legs, as well as sufficient strength to lift the central body mass upward against gravity. Accomplishing this for infants and young children begins with rolling only 5 to 10 degrees from a sidelying position toward a pillow in front that may have an attractive toy on it, or that may be the attractive toy in the form of a stuffed animal. Progress in this direction is measured by using lower and lower support pillows in front until the infant can roll completely onto the abdomen safely and securely.

When this is accomplished, the next step is to start with the body positioned slightly behind sidelying and progress to a lower and lower starting point until the child can roll completely from backlying to pronelying in a comfortable and secure manner. Of course, in order to roll sequentially, the child also has to be able to roll first from sidelying to backlying, then from tummy to backlying. The techniques described above in this chapter can be used to accomplish rolling in addition to the following recommendations.

Recommendations to establish sequential rolling:

- Most babies roll from prone to supine (tummy to back) first. For infants with osteogenesis imperfecta, it is often preferable to work on the sidelying or backlying to tummy roll first because they can control the head more easily in this roll and are less likely to be frightened if the movement occurs quickly.

- It works best to concentrate on rolling in only one direction (right or left) at a time. Begin rolling in the opposite direction only after the first roll is completely achieved.

- Learning to roll requires a few daily opportunities for practice, but generally is a matter of gaining enough strength to complete the task.

- Lack of coordination typically is not a limiting factor in the accomplishment of motor skills, including rolling, for children with osteogenesis imperfecta. When the strength is sufficient, the behavior occurs, although opportunities to practice the skill are necessary.

Prone locomotion or moving while on the tummy is frequently more difficult for children with osteogenesis imperfecta than scooting while sitting. However, fundamental components for movement in prone emerge long before a child typically sits. Given this, and the fact that we can anticipate that prone locomotion will be difficult, why not begin early to help the child increase competence in this skill?

Like scooting in supine, movement in prone is a critical life activity. Everyone needs it, but it's important to recall it represents a *range* of varied locomotor behaviors in this position, not just crawling on hands and knees. We will reintroduce crawling as a locomotor strategy later in this chapter. The goal of this section is to discuss varied prone behaviors that are important for children with osteogenesis imperfecta and how to encourage them.

Prone skills begin to emerge in two positions: 1) when the child begins to take responsibility for holding the head up while facing the caregiver's shoulder, and 2) when lifting and turning the head to clear the face while lying in prone. The former is usually the place to begin by giving the infant opportunities to start holding the head up while fully supported by the adult's hand. Especially at this very early stage of motor development, it is important to keep in mind the *balance between performance and alignment*. One approach is to create the challenge and have the child practice holding the head up regardless of poor alignment, such as the head sagging to one side, from the rational perspective that the neck will get straighter as the muscles get stronger. This can occur, but we suggest an alternative approach, posing this question: Is it intelligent to have the infant practice a skill asymmetrically when it is not necessary to do so? Some types of asymmetry related to osteogenesis imperfecta cannot be changed with exercise. In this case, however, it is a matter of caregiver awareness of the best achievable head position when the baby is performing, beginning with a minimal challenge. This way the infant learns the skill as body segments respond to increasing challenge with practice *in optimal alignment*, in much the same way a concert pianist begins with the right fundamentals to achieve an optimal level of function. The concept of the balance between performance and alignment is applicable to every level of ability for children with osteogenesis imperfecta.

Lifting and turning the head to clear the face while in prone is a lifesaving skill, and a typical neonatal competency. However, infants with osteogenesis imperfecta often cannot do this because of lack of practice, weakness, or body proportions that make this biomechanically very difficult. We described above strategies for achieving this, in particular, using the parent's chest as a support surface and gradually orienting the parent backward on a sofa or chair to increase the challenge for the infant. For this section on prone locomotion, it is important to remember that the joints of the neck and back work together to lift the head and to shift the body weight forward, backward, and sideways. To move this process forward, it may be helpful to position the infant's arms, flexed at the elbows, slightly under the chest, so the infant's chest is resting partially on the forearms. This looks easy, but it is actually quite a challenge for a young infant or weak baby because it changes the baby's weight-bearing pattern on the support surface dramatically. Once the infant has achieved forearm weight-bearing with the head lifted comfortably for very short periods, it's time to focus on encouraging movement.

On the one hand, the ability to lift the head higher and for longer periods, especially linked with forearm support, is a useful skill. However, it's important to consider what is gained versus what is lost when an infant or child is locked into prone position with a wedge or other positioning device under the chest. A careful observer notes that most infants and children learn to dislike this very quickly, possibly because it is hard work, with no escape. This type of device can be useful to elicit weight-bearing in prone in one plane (head up and down), but consider instead strategies that allow the infant the freedom to move in three planes (up and down, forward and backward, sideways).

Adults usually expect prone locomotion to be forward movement, but infants typically begin by pushing backward or sideways. It is usually easiest to begin by encouraging the infant to move sideways in a circle, with the umbilicus as a central axis. For infants with osteogenesis imperfecta, this can be encouraged by placing a desirable object easily within reaching or touching range slightly to the side of the infant's head. Recall that the task must be easy to accomplish initially if you want the baby to succeed, and repeat it. Repetition occurs with presentation of another object that elicits a little more movement to the same side. The weight-shifting and rotation that occur in the body in order to free one arm to reach are complex, so be patient and keep it fun.

Recommendations for encouraging prone locomotion sideways:

- Emphasize moving in only one direction initially until the child has made substantial progress in that direction before starting to work on the opposite direction, then practice going to the right or left side on alternate days.
- If the child has head and neck asymmetry, practice *only* the direction that pulls the head in the desired direction.
- Change toys frequently to elicit the desired behavior.
- Stop when the child is still actively participating, rather than pushing into fatigue or boredom.
- Keep the emphasis on tummy-on-the-floor movement, rather than trying to straighten the arms to push up.

Once the child has made substantial progress going sideways, work begins on moving forward, flat on the tummy, using the same reaching strategies described above, but this time to move forward. In this way *the challenge for arm support is increased gradually and is linked to functionally relevant activities*, as opposed to encouraging static arm extension, which is hard work, and risky.

With increasing practice moving in prone, the child's abdomen may eventually elevate off the support surface (depending on arm strength) for more challenging quadripedal tasks such as *hands-knees crawling*. However, we suggest that the child be given the opportunity to take the lead in this, rather than spending a lot of time trying to elicit this behavior, for the reasons listed below.

Hands-knees crawling:

- A specific child's strength, alignment, time in prone position, and relative body proportions determine skill in hands-knees crawling.
- It is not essential to crawl in order to walk; 12% to 13% of nondisabled children do not crawl before walking.
- It is possible to waste a lot of time trying to accomplish crawling when it is structurally not achievable.
- Children who have fractured in prone in response to challenges they cannot meet may be very reluctant to perform in this position, although they need some form of prone locomotion as a life skill.
- Many children with osteogenesis imperfecta will spend a great deal of time trying to achieve full hip and knee extension (straight hips and knees) throughout their lives.
- Early, intensive focus on hands-knees crawling emphasizes flexed hips and knees, setting up a bias that may be difficult to change later.
- Children who accomplish hands-knees crawling as a successful locomotor strategy should not be discouraged from doing it.
- Transitions into and out of a hands-knees position into sitting, and lying down, may be more appropriate therapeutic goals than hands-knees crawling for children with significant arm weakness or bowing.

Scooting in sitting is a popular way to get around for many children with osteogenesis imperfecta. Like scooting on the back and moving in prone, it is an essential life skill. However, since it is generally easier than locomotion in prone or in supine, children who can sit usually prefer to scoot in sitting. It's obvious that the ability to sit erect and to sit symmetrically (rather than having the head fall to one side) is an essential fundamental to be accomplished before working on scooting in sitting.

Learning to shift the body's weight to one side in order to scoot the opposite leg and pelvis forward is the basis of this behavior. It's easily said, much harder to do. It begins in static ring sitting, legs open, hips fully flexed, knees slightly flexed, by encouraging the child to reach for objects that can be comfortably grasped without making the child fearful of losing balance. The best way to begin is by reaching forward for an object inside the circle made by the child's legs.

As the child becomes more comfortable and skillful with practice in weight-shifting forward and backward, the object to be reached for is placed outside of the circle made by the child's legs. In this way, the child starts to weight-shift laterally. Placing items farther and farther away from the child increases the lateral weight-shift until eventually the child will put down one arm to stabilize the body in order to reach for the object with the other.

Thus, using object placement, and incorporating active reaching, one can elicit weight-shifting of the body's central core in all directions, in a manner that allows the child to improve the skill while in complete control of the task. This is in contrast to putting the child on a ball and moving it sideways to elicit this skill reactively. In the latter case, the child has no control over the situation, does not learn a multilevel skill, and the use of the therapy ball may pose an unnecessary risk since the child is capable of learning to do this actively.

Once the child has learned to weight-shift to unload the opposite side of the body, it is fairly easy to learn to advance the leg and pelvis forward on the unloaded side. The choice then is to scoot using no hands, or to put one hand down on the side the body axis is shifted toward while advancing the opposite leg. Watching the child move in sitting is the best indicator of which method to encourage first. However, it's important to learn to scoot forward, sideways, backward, and in a rotational pattern both with and without hands, since both arms may not always be available following a fracture.

If the child seems to have great difficulty learning to scoot in sitting, the first place to check is for hamstring muscle tightness. Tight muscles on the back of the thighs limit the child's ability to mobilize the pelvis and to extend each knee enough to scoot forward. This may have to be addressed through long sitting or other strategies to gently lengthen the hamstrings before scooting can be accomplished. Use of slippery shorts and a smooth floor rather than a carpet can also progress this skill from a "no go" to a "go." It may be preferable to try this first before elongating the hamstring muscles.

Scooting in sitting:
- Is the basis for the ability to transfer independently into or out of a wheelchair
- Is the gateway to independence for getting into and out of bed, onto or off a couch, onto or off a toilet, up or down stairs, into or out of a bathtub, and into or out of a car
- Can be preliminary to standing and walking for the preambulatory child
- Is useful to interrupt static sitting for extended periods
- Provides a valuable, and cumulative, means of improving cardiopulmonary endurance
- Minimizes the back pain associated with uninterrupted sitting

However, scooting has one drawback. It can contribute to tight hamstrings and the inability to fully extend the knees and hips if the child scoots for most of the day. Scooting or sitting should be balanced with standing or walking, if possible, to provide opportunity for extension of the hips and knees, or at an absolute minimum, with lying prone for at least 30 minutes a day to promote optimal leg and trunk alignment.

Standing is the gateway to walking. Although walking looks like the ability to lift the leg and move the foot forward, it actually depends on the ability to center the body's weight over the *standing* foot while the other foot is in the air. We discussed above the transitions between sitting and standing, and the use of devices to provide supported standing for sustained periods up to 30 to 45 minutes. This section focuses on the relationship between standing and walking. Walking may not be possible for all children with osteogenesis imperfecta, but it is difficult to predict which infants and young children eventually will walk. Why not provide the groundwork to make progress in this domain, and see what happens?

A child who does not have head control, or the ability to sit without support, can be gently raised to a standing position using a supine standing device, but this is not an approach that links to walking. In order to make progress in walking, it is necessary for the child to be able to center the head over the body axis, and to have independent sitting balance. We have discussed earlier in this chapter strategies for addressing asymmetrical head position and improving sitting balance.

To begin work on walking, it is an advantage if the child can transition in and out of sitting and scoot in sitting, but this is often not the case, and it is not necessary to wait for these skills to emerge before starting to work on standing and walking. We discussed above how to begin standing from a sitting position on the caregiver's thigh, or on a low stool, with the child's knees fairly close together and the feet 1 1/2 to 2 inches apart. In particular, we emphasized that the child with osteogenesis imperfecta should not sit with legs open over the caregiver's thigh or on a positioning device that spreads the legs, and then practice standing and sitting with the legs widely apart.

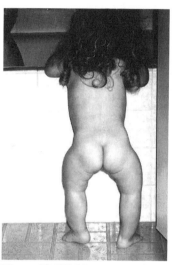

Figure 10. Widely separated legs, in addition to femoral bowing, are a common standing posture for children with osteogenesis imperfecta.

The fact that children with osteogenesis imperfecta tend to have widely separated legs sets them apart from many other children with disabilities who need to widen their base of support in standing (Figure 10). Anticipating this, and in preparation for standing and walking, we emphasized above the important role of sidelying in young infants to help bring their legs together, and for older children, sitting with the knees not touching, but fairly close together, when working on sit-to-stand transitions. We also noted above the preference for parents to avoid carrying infants and young children with osteogenesis imperfecta on their hip with the child's legs widely spread, and to minimize cruising and sidestepping behaviors, encouraging the child to walk forward instead. In spite of these efforts, when the child is ready to begin standing and walking with external support, a position in which the legs are turned outward and widely spread apart often is present when the child attempts standing from a sitting position.

Several factors should be considered before going forward with walking when the legs are widely spaced or the child cannot stand up fully.
    1) Are the hip muscles weak? Children often open the legs in standing to increase stability when weakness is present. Note these are not the muscles that lift the leg; they extend it under the body to support the body's weight over the legs. The *hip extensors* (in the buttocks and back of the thighs) stabilize the legs under the pelvis and link the legs with the back to keep the upper body from falling forward during standing. If these muscles are weak (often in association with weak back muscles), the child's bottom will stick out in back, and it will be difficult or impossible to pull the pelvis in under the body. Exercises done while lying on the tummy to lift one leg at a time, with the knee straight, and without rotating the leg outward, can help transfer this skill to standing. However, many different exercises exist to accomplish this, and it may be helpful to consult a physical therapist to determine the best choices for a particular child.

    Similar to the way hip and back extensors keep the body straight in a forward-to-backward direction, the *hip abductor muscles* work to keep the body level in a side-to-side direction. Located on the outside of the leg at the top of the thigh, they are a short, plate-shaped group of muscles that attach the leg to the pelvis. Their function is to keep the pelvis level, rather than allowing it to tip downward when one leg is lifted. A typical compensation when these muscles are weak on both sides is to space the legs widely, turn them outward, and take short steps. In other words, the compensation during walking for weakness in the hip abductors is not significantly different from that for hip extensors, and in most instances related to osteogenesis imperfecta, both muscle groups are weak. One means of strengthening hip abductors is to position the body in sidelying, both legs straight, and lift the top leg upward and extend it slightly backward. The tendency to roll the pelvis and leg outward and flex the leg forward while lifting (abducting) should be avoided if possible. To be effective, this has to be done on both sides. Of course, there are many other ways to accomplish strengthening this muscle group, as well as the *hip adduc-*

tors, the muscles on the inside of the thigh that hold the legs together under the body during standing.

2) Are the knee muscles weak? The *quadriceps muscles* on the front of the thigh keep the knee extended under the body during standing and work in concert with the *hamstrings muscles* on the back of the thigh to support smooth and stable flexing and extending of the knee and hip during walking. In general, if the child's knee muscles are not strong enough to work against gravity, some type of bracing may be necessary. Sometimes this is done using braces for the foot and ankle, rather than for the whole leg. These muscle groups can also be strengthened in a functional pattern using sit-to-stand activities beginning in a high sitting position with very little hip flexion (the legs are almost extended), then gradually lowering the starting position as the child becomes stronger and more skillful. Lifting the body weight in this way presents the same challenge as putting weights on the legs, but the forces are distributed over many joints, in a functional pattern. It's rare that weakness is only in the knee muscles, and often hip weakness and poor foot alignment are more significant limitations than knee weakness. Thus, analyzing the whole leg and the trunk patterns of movement and weakness is essential to addressing performance problems.

3) Is insufficient joint mobility limiting the ability to fully extend the hips and knees to stand straight enough to walk? This is a completely different problem from weakness, but it is often present at the same time, and the limitations (flexed hips, flexed knees in standing) appear the same as with weakness. The key question is: Can the child extend the hips and knees fully when not standing? Children without osteogenesis imperfecta have 20 to 25 degrees of hip flexion in standing for sometimes up to a year after beginning to walk, so the absence of full hip extension should be expected initially in children with osteogenesis imperfecta. The inability to fully extend the knees is more problematic, and the *first* place to look is at how much time the child is spending in sitting, perhaps in a wheelchair or stroller. This is more problematic for older children, but it needs to be addressed even in young children if much of their awake time is spent sitting with the hips and knees flexed. The good news is that those flexed legs will respond to time spent in prone with legs extended, to straight leg lifts against gravity in prone, and to sit-to-stand exercises with the feet and legs positioned facing forward to activate the muscles that straighten the hips and knees.

4) Is bone and joint malalignment of the legs limiting the ability to stand and walk? Patterns of bowing typically associated with osteogenesis imperfecta are frontal or coronal bowing of the right and left femora (plural for femur), in which the thigh bones curve outward to the side, and sagittal bowing of the right and left tibiae(plural for tibia), in which the largest bone in the calf bows in a forward-backward direction. These bowing patterns are present in varying degree in many infants and children with osteogenesis imperfecta. In general, the presence of lower extremity bowing is not an indication for avoiding standing and walking, with *exceptions as noted below.*

The amount of leg bowing can make it difficult or risky to stand and walk:
- Bowing of 30 degrees or less in the femur or tibia is not an indication to avoid standing or walking.
- Bowing of 30 to 40 degrees is the **pay attention zone.** Consultation with a rehabilitation physician or pediatric orthopedist is necessary to make a decision whether to emphasize standing and walking.
- Bowing of 40 degrees or more is the **zone of risk.** Standing or walking on this bone places the child at risk for spontaneous fracture.
- When bowing exceeds 30 to 40 degrees, the surgeon may recommend osteotomy and intramedullary rodding to straighten the bone and stabilize it by putting in a rod.
- The decision for surgical intervention, and the timing, is made on an individual basis, with many factors to be considered in relation to a specific child.

5) Is weakness or malalignment of the arms limiting the child's ability to stand and walk? Walking appears to be an activity associated with the legs, but children need their arms for balance and stability when beginning to stand and walk. Building arm strength for standing begins with the young infant getting antigravity experience in prone and using the arms to move the body backward, forward, and in a circle. As we discussed above, depending on the severity of weakness and bowing in the arms, prone locomotion may not progress beyond scooting with the abdomen in contact with the surface. However, practice in this position strengthens the same arm muscles that are recruited later to push the body up to standing and to learn walking.

Arm weakness can and should be addressed through exercises for an individual child. Weakness often coexists with significant bowing of the upper arms and/or forearms. This is a challenge requiring ortho-pedic consultation, although surgical intervention may not be appropriate or possible, because of the child's size and the location and amount of bowing. Strictly from the standpoint of walking, the child with weak arms and bowing can gradually be introduced to standing using a supine stander or other standing device, and sometimes can learn to stand with little or no arm support using sit-to-stand exercises. Once standing has been achieved, walker modifications exist to support the child's forearms so that weight-bear-

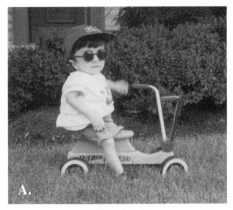

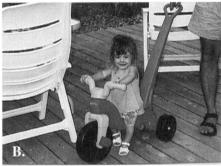

Figure 11. Two types of ride-on toys that can be used preliminary to walking; note that the emphasis is on feet on the ground, rather than pushing the pedals.

ing is spread over the entire length of the forearm. Walker modifications can also be used on a temporary basis to maintain the ability to stand or walk when the child has a fractured arm.

The major factors that limit standing and walking have been discussed in some detail above. Of course, there are other possibilities, and those which promote walking or limit it vary from child to child. Identifying them requires analysis of a child's specific strengths and limitations in order to move for-ward with this new skill.

To the same extent that we recommended earlier in this chapter working on sit-to-stand and standing practice with the feet 1 1/2 to 2 inches apart, emphasis during walking for children with osteogenesis imperfecta is feet straight ahead rather than turned outward. This is a significant departure from

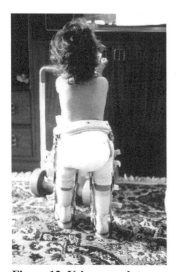

Figure 12. Using a push toy in the same manner a child would use an anterior walker.

a typical developmental progression in which a child pulls up to standing and sidesteps, often in front of the couch or around the coffee table, in a locomotor pattern called cruising. It may not be reasonable to keep a child with osteogenesis imperfecta from cruising with legs widely apart and turned outward, but it is possible to avoid encouraging it, and to substitute an emphasis on walking forward, rather than sideways. This can be done, sometimes after the child has pulled up to standing using the couch or table, by having the child face forward (in the line of progression) and take steps with one hand on the couch or table while the other hand is held by a parent. An alternative is to provide the child with a forward rolling walker (with two wheels to begin), and work on standing with it first, then taking forward steps.

Among the many devices available to encourage walking are ride-on toys (Figure 11), walkers, and push toys (Figure 12), including children's shopping carts. The key concept is what is the best choice for an individual child at a specific level of ability. In general, it's easiest to begin with an anterior or forward rolling walker. Once walking is well established, a reverse or posterior rolling walker may be considered, as pulling the walker from behind can encourage more hip and back extension and promote standing straighter. However, many children with osteogenesis imperfecta are not comfortable without a walker closure in front of them, and the child's sense of security is essential for walking to progress.

Walking is the most challenging of the tasks we have discussed in this chapter. Achieving it may require a clever balancing act on the part of caregivers. The approach is quite different if jump starting the process with long leg braces versus using only orthoses inside the child's shoes to support the midfeet with increasing weight-bearing. In the first case, getting the braces on is the biggest hurdle. The best way to do it is in full supine/backlying, then lifting and placing the child in standing with a walker in front or in the parallel bars during physical therapy. While the child is immediately standing with arm support on the walker or bars, instruction is necessary to learn to weight-shift or lean to one side in order to free or unload the opposite foot to step forward. Promoting this "lean and kick" pattern should make it relatively easy to start taking steps, with the caregiver's hands on the child's pelvis for support and security.

If the child can lean but cannot free and advance the opposite foot, the first place to look is at the bottom of the shoes. Often the textured surface there, designed to avoid falls, creates sufficient friction to make it impossible to advance the foot when wearing long leg braces with the knees extended. An easy fix is to sand off the texture to allow the shoe to slide more easily, and voila! The child walks!

One other important consideration when using long leg braces is to ensure that the child's midfoot (the arch) is well supported inside the foot component of the brace. Frequently this area is overlooked in spite of all the attention to the rest of the brace. If this has occurred, have the orthotist who made the braces modify them so the midfoot arch is well supported before imposing weight-bearing.

Achieving success with long leg braces requires daily effort, for a short time period (5 to 20 minutes), on the part of the parents and the child. There are several strategies, depending on the child, which range from using the braces and a supine stander to accomplish standing first, or, as is more often the case, the child can walk with a little instruction after being placed in standing with a walker or in the parallel bars. With daily practice, skill should improve quickly, and eventually the braces can be cut down to below the knee, and then cut down again until finally only the ankle-foot component remains.

The fact that long leg bracing to promote ambulation is used less often may be related to more consistent early intervention practices for children with osteogenesis imperfecta during their first year of life. Many infants and young children with osteogenesis imperfecta now have anti-gravity head control and the ability to sit within the first year. Short sitting naturally lends itself to weight-bearing on the feet while sitting, thus providing the earliest weight-bearing experience, which then links to standing. We described the progression above, using sit-to-stand exercises to promote a gradual increase in weight-bearing to the child's tolerance.

Once the child can stand with upper extremity support, the same "lean to one side and kick" pattern can be used to transition from standing to walking. Since the weight-bearing is impositional (caregivers are making the decision as to when and how much standing occurs), it is important to support the midfoot arch with orthotic devices in the shoes, which can range from plantar contact only (touching only the bottom of the foot) to above the ankle bones (the malleoli), depending on the child's needs. Supporting the midfoot during weight-bearing is an important consideration even for children who can pull to stand and walk independently, as children with higher motor skill levels often have significant ligamentous laxity and joint hypermobility.

Decisions related to the choice of a gait support device depend on the child's preference and an analysis of the performance level. Children with other diagnoses often progress to crutches, then to canes, before walking with no device. Some children with osteogenesis imperfecta, with the support of their parents, do not wish to use crutches, especially if they have a better gait pattern with a rolling walker than with crutches. Once again, the range of variation is high, and the time spent finding the right means of support is well spent to achieve safe, optimal performance. It's helpful to remember that walking with a gait device requires more effort, and concentration, than walking without one. Thus, for children with osteogenesis imperfecta, promoting independence and reducing reliance on a gait support device are more often a matter of strengthening weak muscles (especially hip abductors, adductors, and extensors, and back extensors) or improving bone and joint alignment, than nagging the child to walk with less support.

Cardiopulmonary Exercise and Endurance

We emphasized above the analysis of infants' and children's skill levels, followed by choices of interventions designed to improve them. The objectives are to increase the child's level of independent function and sense of self-competence in all domains of daily life. Skill is critical to achieving motor performance goals and functional independence, but the ability to perform is equally dependent on endurance and efficiency of effort. This is particularly important for children because the cardiorespiratory system continues to grow and develop in response to the demands placed on it until early adulthood. Thus, special attention must be placed on cardiorespiratory development for children who are not able to move very much on their own. For those who can, the key is to select options which utilize that child's skill level to build endurance.

Improving endurance can be approached at multiple levels in the same manner that we examined skill. For the infant who cannot roll at all, kicking and reaching in supine in the bathtub for several minutes provides a challenge for both skill and endurance, as long as the child is enjoying it. This links nicely, once the child has head control, to wearing an aquatic vest or other support device in the pool or spa in order to play and explore independently.

Once the child can roll, multiple rolls in all directions are a cardiorespiratory challenge as well as a means of improving skill and strength. Scooting in sitting, then walking, are obvious steps in the same direction. But, what about the child approaching age 3 who can sit, but cannot weight-shift in order to scoot, and uses a power chair for locomotion?

Opportunities to give this child a cardiorespiratory challenge include blowing devices that encourage a long, strong exhalation, which is instinctively followed by a large inhalation. This can be achieved in many ways, including blowing Ping-Pong balls across the dining room table to another child or into a basket, or learning to play a recorder as a preschooler, which may later link to playing another wind instrument once in school. One half-hour or more playing in the pool, three to five times a week, is a superb opportunity to build endurance while having fun for a child whose movement is very limited out of the water.

Children who are primarily sitters are at highest risk for developing low cardiopulmonary reserve. Placing expectations on these children to transfer into and out of their chair, rather than the parent picking up and placing the child, is a reasonable place to start to build endurance. The next step to consider is use of a manual chair for short distance travel, using the power chair primarily for long distances.

For children who can stand, beginning to walk in the water has potential benefit for building endurance as well as skill. If need be, this can be done in the bathtub for young children under very close supervision, possibly with a harness, alternating with sitting and blowing bubbles.

For children who can walk, playing in the pool for several hours a few times a week is ideal, especially if linked with singing or playing a musical instrument in an educational setting during the week. *Walking every day, even for only a few minutes*, is the way to maintain and improve this skill, and to build endurance specific to this task.

Thus, it is obvious that building endurance is an essential part of any skill development program. If it is perceived as a burden, most children and parents will gradually stop doing it. In contrast, creative thinking to identify recreational opportunities to build skill and endurance, rather than just "doing exercises," is often more successful and reinforces a balanced life style that is fun and sustainable.

How Much Time for Intervention?

In general, total time per day allocated for intervention activities varies from 15 minutes to 1 hour, although positioning strategies for infants should occur throughout the day. Time varies significantly according to the needs and general activity level of the child, date of the most recent fracture, and the composition of the family. In general, very short sessions integrated into the day, as described in the guidelines above, are more effective for infants and younger children. Even for older children, practicing walking for 5 minutes every day will accomplish much more than doing this for 1 1/2 hours once a week in therapy.

It's often helpful to focus on achieving one specific goal at a time. Consistent effort, within the child's tolerance, can result in better performance within days, although complex skills may require weeks or months of effort. For example, gaining better head control by lifting a young infant's shoulders, caregiver's hands behind the shoulders, to elicit neck muscle contraction in supine two to four times, following diaper changes, usually generates results in days or weeks. Effort here will contribute to better head control in rolling, sitting, and standing months later. However, if the challenge is too difficult, or if it occurs too often, the baby will go on strike, and no longer respond. Thus, parents and other caregivers must pay attention to the needs and behavior of the child, at any age, and be prepared to change the program in order to maintain the child's interest and ability to derive satisfaction from accomplishment.

Summary points:
- Infants with osteogenesis imperfecta can benefit from early, varied, positioning experiences to lay the groundwork for later movement skills.

- Early positioning and movement interventions work best if incorporated, in small doses, into the natural flow of caregiving activities during the day.
- Motor development progresses from static body positions to movements between these positions, then to achieving locomotor capability in backlying, prone, sitting, and standing.
- The environment should be structured to have fun whenever possible and to build the child's sense of accomplishment.
- Use warm water to learn early kicking and during recovery from fractures or surgery.
- Provide positive feedback to the child that describes what occurred, and keep the emphasis on what the child has accomplished rather than on pleasing the parent.
- Wait for the child to do it (for instance, dressing).
- Network with parents, educators, and medical professionals to make choices for an individual child from the wide range of equipment options available.
- Consider medical professionals, including physicians, nurses, and therapists, as well as educators, as part of the team devoted to the needs of the child. If the teamwork is not working, parents may have to take the initiative to communicate this and help seek solutions.

CHAPTER THREE

STRATEGIES FOR CHILDREN

*Improving strength and endurance while
promoting optimal alignment and joint mobility*

Holly Lea Cintas, PT, PhD

Goals for middle childhood (ages 4 to 12 years), a period of partnering:
- Improve the child's strength, stamina, and general mobility level
- Monitor body alignment in relation to support devices, such as wheelchairs and walkers, to identify and minimize asymmetry
- Develop strategies with parents and children, working together, to ensure that most of the day is not spent sitting in the same position in a wheelchair
- Take time in the short run to allow the child to practice a task in order to achieve independent function in the long run
- Reduce the risk of obesity
- Achieve independent dressing, toileting, and bathing or make significant progress toward them
- Have fun being active

Introduction

Infants and children younger than 4 years of age need physical assistance and emotional guidance to complete their day. As the child matures, the parent's role shifts increasingly from doing for the child to doing with the child. Ideally, the objectives achieved during middle childhood build on strategies initiated earlier. For example, nurturing the infant's and young child's interest in helping take socks and shoes or shirt and pants on and off should result in complete or nearly complete independence in these activities during middle childhood. A 5-year-old child who cannot sit or stand can reasonably be expected to put on underwear and take it off while lying down. Of course, there are days when children need help getting dressed in order to get to school on time, but to the extent possible, the focus should be on gaining long-term independence for daily life activities. Even though it takes longer for the young child to get in and out of bed independently, possibly requiring assistive devices to complete this, or to transfer from a wheelchair to a desk chair in school, allowing time for the child to accomplish this independently is an important investment in the child's future.

Developing Self-Competence and Setting Realistic Expectations for Performance

Achieving optimal performance for any person, including a child with osteogenesis imperfecta, is the result of a finely tuned balancing act. If the bar is set too high, if expectations are beyond what is perceived as reasonable, even an infant will give up quickly, developing a pattern of repeated failure. To avoid this requires balancing the realities of now and later. On the one hand, the long-term goal for the child with osteogenesis imperfecta is to develop fully independent function in all life domains using adaptive devices as needed. On the other, the key to getting there is setting goals so that the child usually succeeds in attaining them and often exceeds them.

To the extent possible, the child's achieving the target behavior should be the outcome and its own reward. The sense of accomplishment associated with it is what counts, rather than the amount of praise the child receives for doing it. In this way children take increasing responsibility for mastering the environment. They gain life skills in the course of doing it, and learn to achieve for the sake of achievement, rather than constantly acting in response to the burden of pleasing others. The challenge of partnering for parents is to offer praise and share the joy of accomplishment with one's child, while at the same time nurturing increasing levels of independence in a way that can be sustained by the child (Figure 1).

The Cyclic Nature of Performance in Osteogenesis Imperfecta

It is important to consider the balance between long-term goals and short-term accomplishments discussed above as a developmental process. However, fractures and surgical procedures associated with osteogenesis imperfecta

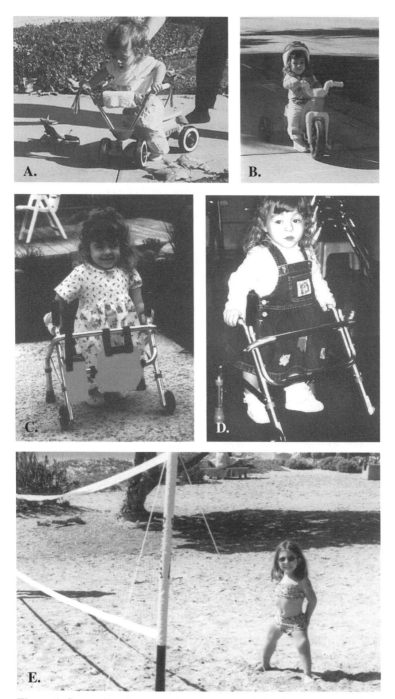

Figure 1. Succeeding in small steps to accomplish a long-range goal.

often result in losses in independent function that can be physically and psychologically demoralizing for the whole family. One approach is to simply accept that performance is going to be cyclic (Figure 2). Under the best circumstances, there are going to be ups and downs. Another approach is to recognize what can be done under current circumstances; for instance, a child in a spica cast can blow Ping-Pong balls across a low table, aiming them into a basket, to maintain or improve cardiopulmonary reserve. Singing or playing a recorder also addresses this goal. The same child can be doing exer-

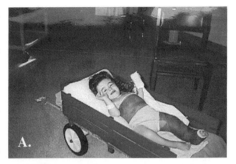

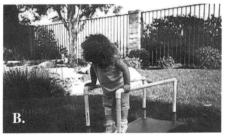

Figure 2. Performance in osteogenesis imperfecta is cyclic.

cises with the arms, especially reaching upward toward the ceiling one arm at a time while lying on the back, possibly using a small weight or a small can of tomato paste. Lifting the head in an effort to tuck the chin activates the neck and abdominal muscles, although repetitive sit-up exercises in the spica are not recommended because of muscular linkages between the abdominal muscles, pelvis, and legs. Once out of the spica, the best place for the child to start moving again is in warm water, simply letting the child explore and do what is comfortable in terms of movement. Daily opportunities for 2 to 3 weeks in a warm swimming pool or spa are a good choice for this, but it can be accomplished during 20 to 30 minutes in the bathtub if necessary.

If one arm or leg is immobilized because of fracture or surgery, this does not mean the rest of the body is off limits for exercise or activity, or that physical therapy has to be cancelled during this period. Common sense reigns in this situation. Exercises that could produce pain in the fractured extremity are obviously unacceptable. For example, challenging abdominal exercises will activate the leg and shoulder muscles and should be avoided if the child has a fractured humerus (upper arm) or femur (upper leg). On the other hand, forced expiration using blow bottles and activities like playing a recorder or singing require abdominal effort without the risk of shoulder or leg pain.

Children who have had spinal surgery for scoliosis require much more vigilance in terms of safe exercise choices. Since the arms and legs are suspended from the body by muscles attaching them to the trunk, challenging exercises for any extremity can be painful and undesirable after spinal surgery. In general, movements of the arms or legs, one at a time, that are not uncomfortable are acceptable. Progression from rolling the body to sidelying as if it were a log, followed by pushing up to sitting from sidelying, and eventually sitting up from backlying (usually with a back brace on) must be made in close consultation with the orthopedic surgeon who performed the surgery and the physical therapist working with that child. Every effort should be made to ensure a smooth and uneventful recovery. It is not a no pain, no gain situation. Children with osteogenesis imperfecta may require a slower, more conservative return to upright standing and walking after spinal surgery than children with scoliosis only. Once the child can safely travel with minimal discomfort, opportunities to begin moving again in warm water are helpful and should be comfortable rather than exhausting.

Identifying and Focusing on Objectives

Parents and their children frequently know what they want in terms of physical performance or independence, but where to begin the progression to achieve it may not be clear. So many things are wanted or needed that it's hard to know where to begin. It is valuable to focus on one objective at a time, especially one that is meaningful for the child and useful for the parents in terms of increasing the child's independence. The chances of achieving it are much greater if everyone on the team is focused on this objective, including the physical and occupational therapists in the school setting or other environments, the adaptive or regular physical education teacher, and the child's classroom teacher. Of course, parameters vary according to whether the child is in preschool or elementary or middle school, but the idea of working together to help the child move forward is applicable to all settings, including day care.

With respect to scheduling specific therapeutic exercises in a child's day, needs vary according to the child's interests and level of function. In general, children who are primarily sitting will benefit from time spent out of the wheelchair standing or lying prone to avoid losing the ability to completely straighten the hips and knees (Figure 3). Complemented by daily exercises to strengthen the back muscles and those that extend the hips and knees, this approach can support the child's continuing ability to bear weight while standing and possibly result in walking. For the

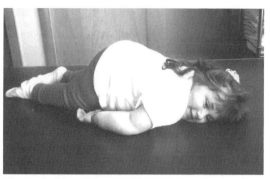

Figure 3: Pronelying as a way of extending the hips and knees; supplemented by exercises in prone position, this is an important alternative to many hours of sitting.

child with minimal or no difficulty walking, exercise interventions can be focused on obtaining the best possible body alignment with growth and developing strength and endurance through recreational pursuits.

Physical and occupational therapy in school is designed to ensure that children with disabilities benefit maximally from their educational setting and gain independence in life skills like their classmates. Thus, the target emphasis is improving functional skills and achieving independent function. The child's classroom teacher, physical education teacher, and personal care aide are key players on this team. However, the approach to achieving improved performance varies according to the state and the school district. Some parents supplement school therapy with additional private therapy visits after a period of inactivity or immobilization following surgery or fracture. Many parents have reported success with consistent emphasis on physical or occupational therapy-related activities during the school year, replaced by swimming for several hours daily during the summer.

Building a Better Back and Trunk

Limitations in joint mobility, strength, or alignment are readily apparent in the legs and arms. Thus, the tendency is to focus efforts on improving the range of motion and alignment of specific joints of the arms and legs and strengthening the muscles. These efforts are important, but back alignment and strength are often overlooked in this process. Recall that the arms and legs literally hang from the trunk. Muscle linkages that connect the trunk, shoulders, and hips stabilize the body's central core so the shoulder and hip muscles can pull from a secure base in order to move the arms and legs. Thus, a strong trunk (back plus front) is not only an advantage in terms of alignment, it is essential to achieve optimal performance of the arms and legs.

Children with osteogenesis imperfecta are at risk for developing neck and back asymmetries, such as torticollis, scoliosis, kyphosis, and lordosis. Torticollis, the tendency of the head to lean to one side, was discussed in Chapter 2 in relation to infants, with emphasis on the importance of remediating the condition early and aggressively by means of exercises and positioning. Early asymmetry in the back, leaning to one side, can occur after a young child has fractured one arm and is using the other arm exclusively for scooting or for transfers into and out of a wheelchair. This is usually temporary, but should be monitored. It can be addressed by encouraging the child to scoot with the legs only, or by reaching above the head one arm at a time as an exercise, stretching the arm as "long" as possible to fully extend the back. The time line for doing this depends on the status of the fractured arm, and if the child is consistently leaning to the right, for example, the decision may be to reach and stretch with only the right arm to selectively elongate that side of the body.

It is often the case in early, temporary asymmetry that the child begins to develop a habit of sitting to one side, with more weight on one buttock than the other. This is subtle and frequently undiscovered until it is well established, but it should be anticipated when the alignment of the trunk above the pelvis is asymmetrical. In addition to reaching overhead to elongate the back and scooting with no arms, it can be useful to use exercise strategies that elicit weight-shifting of the pelvis in the opposite direction onto the other buttock. These are developed for an individual child with a physical therapist because they require fine tuning to achieve the desired outcome: a level pelvis in sitting.

Scoliosis, a curving of the spine sideways, can be behavioral or structural. In the former, known as *functional scoliosis*, the child's spine is curved, but the curve is not fixed and can be reduced through a change in body position. In contrast, the curve is fixed in *structural scoliosis*. It cannot be changed by moving the body or extending the spine. A single C-curve in the midportion or thoracic area of the back is most common. A compensatory second curve can also be present in the lower back or lumbar region, creating an S-curve.

Exactly what causes spinal asymmetries in osteogenesis imperfecta cannot be established with certainty, but it is likely that several factors contribute. These may include abnormal bone growth, muscle weakness, joint hyperflexibility, and ligamentous laxity. Poor body alignment during sustained sitting, especially associated with many uninterrupted hours in a wheelchair, and different leg lengths resulting in a nonlevel pelvis during standing are also potential factors contributing to scoliosis and other spinal abnormalities.

Interventions for scoliosis are anticipatory or reactive. In anticipation of spinal asymmetry, vigilance on the part of all caregivers, especially those in a healthcare setting, can be effective. Identifying and remediating torticollis in the infant or young child have already been described. For the child who consistently sits or scoots while positioned over one buttock, strategies to shift weight-bearing to the other side in order to elongate the back on the short side and level the pelvis can be considered. If scooting or sitting on one side only is short term, for example, associated with a fracture, it is probably not a concern for long-term alignment. However, multiple fractures of the same arm or leg can lead to a pattern of trunk asymmetry that should be anticipated and addressed.

Careful attention to the child's alignment in the wheelchair is an important anticipatory strategy because the child's body changes, but the wheelchair remains the same as it was when last modified. Appropriate seat and back cushions, the child's alignment in the chair, and the amount of time the child sits in the chair are factors as important as any exercise program. Wheelchairs or strollers with sling (nonfirm) seats are inexpensive, lightweight, and appropriate for short distances, but often the child's pelvis is not level in this type of seat. Ironically, custom seating systems, the opposite extreme in terms of expense and control, can also contribute to poor back alignment in some children with osteogenesis imperfecta.

With the exception of those with severe trunk malalignment who cannot sit comfortably without a custom seating system, children with osteogenesis imperfecta generally do better with a semifirm or firm, flat, seat cushion and back cushion. Not only do these allow the child to shift and move over the seat, but they encourage independent transfers into and out of the wheelchair. A scooped-out contour seat may be the best choice for a child with a neurological disability for whom trunk alignment is critical to hand function, but a curved seat makes it more difficult for a child with osteogenesis imperfecta to transfer into and out of the chair. Also, the same stability provided by a contour seat for the child with poor head and trunk control results in the child with osteogenesis imperfecta sitting in exactly the same place in the chair for long periods, which can become a source of chronic back pain.

One of the most important interventions to minimize the potential for back pain, and to promote good back and hip alignment, is to ensure that the child does not spend the whole school day sitting in the wheelchair. At a minimum of once during the school day the child should get out of the chair, with help if necessary, to stand, walk, or lie in prone with hips and knees extended, perhaps on the couch in the nurse's office, for 20 minutes. If this is not possible, standing to transfer from the wheelchair into a school desk chair may also help avoid the back pain associated with many hours of sitting.

Although contour back and seat cushions can be problematic for children with osteogenesis imperfecta, modifications can be made to flat cushions for comfort, to improve alignment, and to accommodate growth. Attaching a lumbar support for the low back to a flat back cushion or adding lateral (side) trunk supports are two among many possible modifications that are easily adjusted to improve upright alignment. A rear head (occipital) support is essential for safe wheelchair travel in a bus or van, but is rarely necessary in other situations and limits rather than encourages movement for children with osteogenesis imperfecta. A harness system with wide straps for highway travel can be an important consideration relative to the child's size and weight.

Falls out of the wheelchair are problematic. The device intended to ensure staying in the chair in the event of a tip forward is a seat belt, or a harness, which works only if used. Therefore, the first line of intervention to avoid a fall out of the chair is to train children to *buckle up as soon as they get into the chair.* One seat belt system useful for individuals with osteogenesis imperfecta is an airplane-type seat belt that is secure when closed, but the belt is easily introduced into the buckle. If the child cannot open and close a click-closure buckle and requires help each time, this increases the potential for dependence and a lower activity level. Similarly, Velcro closure belts, although easy to open and close, do not have an alarm system to alert the user when they will fail with repeated use. Some children and parents prefer a harness system for everyday transport. The key concept to remember is that if it becomes an ordeal to get into or out of the wheelchair, transfers will happen less frequently. Although a harness can be a useful safety device for some children with osteogenesis imperfecta, especially in a car, it is rarely needed to compensate for trunk weakness and has little or no meaningful influence on alignment.

To return to our discussion of spinal asymmetry, vigilance to identify early evidence of asymmetry includes the potential for *leg length discrepancy*, another source of pelvic tilting or obliquity. Depending on fracture history, bowing, or unequal leg growth, one leg can be longer than the other. This can develop within a short period in osteogenesis imperfecta. Which leg is longer can also change within a few months. The key is to identify a leg length difference, measure it, and then decide what to do about it.

Measurement of leg lengths lying down can give some indication of a difference, but the major influence of leg length difference on the pelvis and back occurs in standing. Thus, it is essential to do this measurement in a standing position for children who stand or walk. This is easily done at the physician's or physical therapist's office using boards of different thicknesses under the foot of the short leg to see what height levels the pelvis. Once the determination is made, a lift of up to 1/4-inch thickness can usually go in the shoe; anything larger is attached to the bottom of the shoe. An orthopedic or specialty shoestore can do this with a prescription from a physician. A bracemaker (orthotist) can also attach the lift, but generally it costs more than if done at a shoestore. Sometimes children are annoyed at having to wear a lift, but they often agree if time is taken to explain why it is essential to level the pelvis, and that the lift may not be required for long-term alignment.

Exercises that elongate and extend the trunk to improve posture and strength can be considered an anticipatory strategy in relation to scoliosis. These include overhead reaching with one arm at a time to exert a pulling or traction force on the back. The idea is to make the arm as "long" as possible, extending the arm directly toward the ceiling while positioning it close to the ear, rather than reaching forward. Daily (Monday to Friday) repetitions of a minimum of 20 and up to 100 are not that much effort and can have a noticeable effect on the child's posture in sitting and standing. For younger children, reaching up to touch a tape or string across a doorway while alternating arms and counting to 20 can be sufficient motivation to do overhead reaching daily. Throwing small balls over a high net and tossing a basketball in a manner that elicits full arm extension above the head are other possibilities for older children.

Suspending the body's weight on "monkey bars" with straight elbows (not pull-ups) under close parental supervision is still another means of elongating and strengthening the back. For older children, swimming provides strengthening as well as extension and elongation of the back, especially if the emphasis is on back crawl. Even for young children, depending on their level of ability, swimming also can be effective to achieve strengthening and back elongation.

Kyphosis often responds well to the same exercise strategy. A slight rounding of the upper back is normal, but an ***increased thoracic kyphosis*** refers to an exaggerated rounded upper back with shoulders forward. Although pulling the shoulder blades back and together while sticking out the chest would seem to be the obvious choice to remedy this, the reality is that most children (and adults) hate this and won't do it consistently. In contrast, reaching directly overhead as a stretch pulls each shoulder backward and extends the upper back as effectively as pulling the shoulder blades together, but it's more fun and tolerable. It is usually more effective to extend one arm at a time over the head. However, a two-arm stretch can certainly be put into the mix for some variety, especially if the child is suspended from an overhead bar under close adult supervision. Evaluating sustained sitting time in the wheelchair, especially while leaning over a desk, and increasing daily activity levels out of the chair are also crucial interventions to minimize kyphosis. A small, minimally intrusive lumbar support in the wheelchair can often have an impressive effect on reducing kyphosis.

Lordosis is the term used for describing the scoop or curve in the lower back. It is naturally exaggerated in children less than 2 years of age. However, it becomes a source of concern when the curve increases significantly in association with long-term sitting and/or the inability to fully extend the hips during standing or in pronelying. This is related to shortening of the hip flexor muscles joining the legs to the pelvis in front, and weakness of the hip extensor muscles joining the legs to the pelvis in back. *Increased lumbar lordosis* is best addressed in children with osteogenesis imperfecta through exercise, increased activity levels out of the chair, and positioning.

Exercises for lordosis focus on two areas:
- Increasing abdominal strength and flattening the back through crunches or semi-sit-ups (starting in 45 degrees of sitting)
- Increasing the strength of the hip extensor muscles (and the length of the hip flexor muscles) to bring the pelvis under the chest in standing

There are additional benefits to increasing abdominal strength and flexing the trunk (bending the body at the hips) beyond flattening the back. Effort and improved performance in this area make it easier and faster to sit up from lying down, a life skill that can be very challenging for some children with osteogenesis imperfecta.

Increasing the length of the hip flexor muscles, and concurrently, the strength of the hip extensor muscles, requires analysis of the source of the hip flexor shortness. We will elaborate on this below in relation to limited joint mobility. Here it is sufficient to say that *stretching to gain muscle length is usually futile unless the source of the shortening is identified and an effort is made to modify the factors contributing to it*. In the case of tight hip flexors in middle childhood and adolescence, the body's adaptation to long periods of uninterrupted sitting is hip (and often knee) flexor tightness. This tightness, combined with weak hip extensors and prolonged static sitting, is a behavioral factor linking to lumbar lordosis that can be modified through position changes and exercise. Infants and young children, in contrast, gradually increase hip flexor length with growth and activity over the first 2 years. Thus, increased lumbar lordosis is not abnormal in young children and recent walkers. However, even young children with osteogenesis imperfecta are at risk for hip flexor tightness, hip extensor weakness, and increased lumbar lordosis if they spend much of their time in uninterrupted sitting.

Obesity often coexists with increased lumbar lordosis in children with osteogenesis imperfecta, although there is no evidence that they are related. Both, however, respond to increased activity levels. The gradual development of increased lumbar lordosis and weight gain signals that action be taken. This usually means breaking up long periods of sitting in the wheelchair with land exercise, swimming, standing, or walking. If the child gets out of the wheelchair to stand momentarily only once an hour, this makes a significant difference compared with uninterrupted sitting for many hours. For children who cannot stand, lying in prone for 20 minutes per day at school, supplemented by a half hour at home provides the back and hip extension leading to better pelvic alignment. If during this time the child rolls into and out of prone in both directions, this muscular effort not only reinforces prone alignment and strengthens the hip extensors, but helps increase the heart rate and activity level, and burns calories, for a child who is not able to stand.

We discussed above anticipatory strategies and interventions in relation to spinal curvature in the frontal (scoliosis) and sagittal (kyphosis and lordosis) planes of the body. Kyphosis and lordosis generally respond to exercise, increased activity, and positioning, but sometimes our best efforts are not sufficient to stop the progression of scoliosis. In addition to the anticipatory strategies we described above, the most important intervention for scoliosis is a baseline x-ray of the spine at the first sign of asymmetry. This baseline assessment is essential to determine the presence of a curve, and, over time, whether it is progressing and at what rate. Children without osteogenesis imperfecta are often fitted with a back brace when a scoliotic curve measures 20 to 30 degrees. However, the effectiveness of this brace depends on sustained pressure against the bones of the chest, so this approach may not be appropriate for all children with osteogenesis imperfecta. Aggressive exercise strategies to elongate the back and strengthen the trunk, described above in this chapter, are typically the focus of intervention for children with osteogenesis imperfecta, rather than bracing, but there are exceptions depending on the needs of a specific child.

A scoliotic curve of 40 or more degrees can be an indication to consider evaluation and surgical intervention by a pediatric orthopedist who specializes in spinal surgery. Surgical intervention for scoliosis, like bracing, is based on a consideration of many factors relating to the individual needs of a specific child. After surgery, the first interventions are gradual mobilization, beginning with log rolling from the back to the side in order to sit up, and gentle arm and leg exercises that do not challenge the back muscles to cause pain. Children with osteogenesis imperfecta may not be able to tolerate the often aggressive rate of progression to sitting or standing after spinal surgery indicated for children without the condition. It can be helpful to discuss the planned progression to the upright position with the surgeon before the surgery. Once at home, if possible, the ideal place to begin moving again is in a warm pool, spa, or bathtub, where the child makes the decisions to gradually increase movement at a comfortable, self-controlled pace.

Chest Realities: Scoliosis, Pectus Carinatum, and Pectus Excavatum

Back strength and alignment were discussed above in the context of the trunk, emphasizing its stabilizing role for movement of the arms and legs. The chest, in contrast, is designed for maximal mobility, relatively independent of the arms. The pectoral muscles on the front of the shoulder attach to the sternum, or breastbone, and the neck muscles elevate the clavicle, or collarbone, but these muscles generally do not influence movement of the chest unless they are called on to assist in respiration, an extremely rare event in osteogenesis imperfecta. The abdominal muscles, in contrast, attach on the lower ribs and play an important role in activities requiring forced expiration, such as coughing, singing, playing a recorder or oboe, yelling, and laughing. The abdominal muscles insert at the other end on the pelvis, spanning the abdomen to support the abdominal contents, and to provide the power to sit up from lying down.

In the same way that bones in osteogenesis imperfecta grow creatively and don't follow the rules in the legs and back, the bones of the chest can develop according to their own plan. This can occur in the ribs in association with scoliosis. Sometimes the vertebral bodies, the central section of each bone in the spine, rotate as part of the spinal curvature, and when this occurs, the ribs attached to those vertebral bodies rotate as well. This creates a protrusion, usually consisting of several ribs, on the front or back of the chest or both. Rib rotation and associated thoracic asymmetry may be early evidence of scoliosis, and can be considered an indication for baseline x-ray of the spine.

More common chest deformities associated with osteogenesis imperfecta also include the ribs, but they are apparent on the front of the chest, at the sternum or breastbone. *Pectus carinatum* refers to an elevated sternum in which the front of the chest is high, and the whole thorax, even including the lower ribs, is high in relation to the length of the trunk. In *pectus excavatum*, the sternum is depressed and the chest has a scooped out appearance, especially over the lower sternum. In general, the thorax does not appear as high-riding as in pectus carinatum and is longer in relation to the entire length of the trunk. Once again, it is likely that these chest deformities are multifactorial; no single cause can be readily identified.

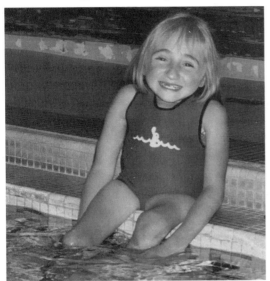

Figure 4: Swimming, or just playing in the water, is an excellent choice of activity to build endurance as well as strength.

Ironically, pectus carinatum and pectus excavatum, or some combination of the two in the same child, may have little impact on respiratory function. However, in conjunction with low activity levels and obesity, they may be an additional factor limiting respiratory function. To the extent possible, and within the child's comfort level, children with pectus carinatum should have prone experience to promote the development of increased respiratory capacity in the back of the chest, as well as the opportunity to develop prone locomotion skills. This is much easier to begin in infancy but is still possible to accomplish in older children with short intervals and sustained effort.

Interventions to improve cardiopulmonary function and *endurance* in children with osteogenesis imperfecta are based on the fact that the thorax and lungs continue to develop in response to demand until early adulthood. Thus, active children who are rolling, scooting, swimming, moving from sitting to standing, or walking are developing heart and lung capacity and the muscles of respiration at the same time they are using other muscles. In addition, these activities contribute to more efficient function of the skeletal muscles participating in the activities (Figure 4).

For the child with limited independent motor skills, perhaps because of multiple surgeries over several months, a program of singing instruction and choral participation, or playing a wind instrument, such as a recorder, piccolo, flute, or clarinet, might be considered. A younger child might enjoy and would benefit from any blowing activities, such as games with Ping-Pong balls, candles under supervision, or blow bottles.

A frequent emphasis in this chapter has been to find ways to interrupt sustained sitting in a wheelchair. Although out-of-chair activities are preferred, *wheelchair push-ups* in which the child pushes on the arm rests to lift the body off the seat can strengthen the arms and trunk and improve endurance in some children. However, given the proportion of the size of the arms to the size of the body, laxity of the elbow joint, and bowing in the arms, this should not be considered a primary source of strengthening.

Joint Mobility: Too Much or Too Little and What to Do About It

Range of motion or movement of the joints varies widely in children with osteogenesis imperfecta. Evidence of hyperflexibility is easily apparent in the knees and elbows, which can be hyperextended and appear double-jointed. Some parents report that their children put their feet up over the head while sleeping. Thus, *many joints can be hyperflexible*, but it is more obvious in certain body areas. While one might not initially focus on hyperflexibility in the ankles and feet, this area is frequently the most problematic in terms of the impact on function for children who stand or walk.

Since most of the muscles of the ankle and foot are in the lower leg, many bones in the foot and ankle are dependent on ligaments and tendons to hold them in place and to provide the "bounce" in the foot that allows us to shift our relatively large bodies smoothly from foot to foot. Laxity of the ligaments and tendons of the foot often results in flattening or loss of the midfoot arch during weight-bearing. This can occur in conjunction with laxity in the hindfoot (the subtalar joint) so that the heel bone (the calcaneus) appears to sway outward (eversion) in addition to flattening of the midfoot. Children with osteogenesis imperfecta can walk on these severely pronated feet for years without complaining and sometimes do so to avoid wearing orthotic devices. However, the bounce described above is lost, foot malalignment increases with malalignment of adjacent joints, and the walking pattern becomes increasingly less efficient.

The challenge is to maintain foot and ankle alignment with increasing growth and upright activity. Several approaches can be considered. Children who are pulling up to stand by themselves can benefit from "free feet," meaning no shoes or soft shoes to avoid limiting activity of the foot so an arch develops in the same way as in children without hyperflexibility. The key to this approach is an awareness of the child's foot alignment over time. A low or no arch is typical for all new standers and walkers. However, if it appears that the heel bone is beginning to sway inward, or more commonly in osteogenesis imperfecta, outward, it may be wise to evaluate this child for an orthotic device to balance weight-bearing on the inside and outside of the foot.

Some active standers go up on their toes, a source of concern for parents and caregivers. Although this can be problematic for children with cerebral palsy and other neurological diagnoses, this is rarely the case for children with osteogenesis imperfecta. Toe standing or walking is usually of short duration, and going up on the forefoot by elevating the heel bone actually helps to promote arch development. Given the ligamentous laxity and joint hyperflexibility associated with osteogenesis imperfecta, it is particularly important to avoid passive stretching exercises to gain more dorsiflexion (flexing the foot upward toward the leg). Forcing the foot upward usually stretches the connective tissues on the bottom of the foot that support the arch, rather than the much larger and stronger Achilles tendon. Increased range of motion can be readily gained through functional activities and a careful analysis of what factors are contributing to the limited range. Often, reestablishing weight-bearing is an effective way to increase the length of the Achilles tendon. However, if it is essential to stretch passively to gain dorsiflexion, this should be done by manually depressing the heel while fully supporting the arch, so that the stretch is applied specifically to the shortened Achilles tendon.

Another approach merits consideration for children who are not pulling up into standing on their own. Young children without osteogenesis imperfecta, and some with it, spend many months of practice before accomplishing active standing and walking. They gain foot, ankle, knee, and hip strength and alignment during the process, demonstrated by the fact that they achieve standing independently. Nonstanding children with osteogenesis imperfecta are appropriately given experience in standing with caregiver assistance, supine standers, or braces to provide opportunities to become stronger and to accelerate their motor skills. However, these are passive standing strategies in which the child does not control the weight-bearing as in active standing. Since this weight-bearing is imposed, there are advantages to supporting the midfeet as weight-bearing is applied. Means of doing this are discussed elsewhere (Chapters 2 and 7) in the context of orthotic devices (in-shoe supports) or orthoses (braces).

The same considerations apply to older children who haven't been standing for several weeks or months while recovering from a fracture or surgery. Their muscles and other soft tissues often lack strength and resilience. They may also be shortened and stiff because of lack of movement and will respond to the gradual introduction of weight-bearing to provide gentle elongation of the muscles and soft tissues as well as loading of the bone. Reestablishing standing should include an evaluation of foot alignment in supported standing and, if necessary, a consideration of midfoot and hindfoot support in the form of off-the-shelf or custom orthotic devices for children without braces. For children with braces, careful evaluation of the midfoot section of the brace is suggested to ensure it offers adequate support during the reintroduction of standing.

Limited range of motion in the foot and ankle is relatively unusual. If ankle motion is painful or very limited in the absence of fracture or soft tissue injury, tibial rod migration downward into the joint space should be considered. Occasionally, limited dorsiflexion (foot up) can occur with moderate to severe bowing of the tibia in the sagittal (forward to backward) plane. It's obvious that stretching will not overcome this bony limitation, only realignment of the tibia resolves it. More often, limited dorsiflexion is the result of the absence of weight-bearing, which allows the Achilles tendon to shorten. This is frequently resolved in osteogenesis imperfecta with the gradual reintroduction of weight-bearing, using heel wedges initially and midfoot support for comfortable standing. This functional stretching is preferable to passive manual stretching of the bottom of the foot. For nonstanding children with limited dorsiflexion, the same approach can be used for weight-bearing on the feet in a wheelchair: elevating the heels initially, then gradually reducing the size of the wedges until the feet rest comfortably flat on the footplate.

The nature of joints is to join. We started this section with a discussion of hyperflexibility in the foot and ankle because it is easily overlooked and its subtle progression has important functional consequences for standing and walking. However, it is impossible to consider the foot and ankle in isolation from the knee. They share a large weight-bearing bone, the tibia, which often takes its own creative direction in terms of sagittal plane bowing. The fibula, the smaller bone next to the tibia on the outside of the leg, is not a weight-bearing bone at the ankle or knee, but is an attachment site for muscles controlling movement at the knee and ankle. Like the tibia, the fibula can also grow according to its own plan, sometimes curling around the tibia. Thus, foot, ankle, and knee alignment is much more than a matter of ligament or tendon laxity. Many factors contribute to the complex picture of hyperflexibility, joint range of motion, and bone and joint alignment. Hyperflexibility in the knee frequently presents in a dynamic manner as *hyperextension*, which occurs in the sagittal plane. This often responds to strengthening exercises focused on sit-to-stand activities.

Sit-to-stand exercises to improve hyperextension of the knee are designed to strengthen the following structures:
• Quadriceps muscles on the front of the leg
• Hamstrings and adductor muscles on the back and inside of the leg
• Tendons and ligaments crucial to knee stability and alignment

The objective of sit-to-stand exercises is to increase strength and to balance it across the joint, through the whole arc of movement of the knee, without hyperextending the knee. The child begins by sitting on a high surface (with 30 to 45 degrees of knee flexion), then stands without completely extending the knee, approximately 5 to 10 degrees short of full knee extension. After 5 to 20 repetitions in this position, this is repeated from a lower sitting surface (45 to 60 degrees of knee flexion), then repeated again from an even lower surface (60 to 75 degrees of knee flexion). The lowest sitting surface should not exceed 90 degrees of knee and hip flexion, often called a squat, as this puts an undesirable amount of stress on the knee ligaments and tendons. This exercise often helps the child gain insight into when the knees are hyperextended during standing and walking, and it is far more effective than constant reminders not to hyperextend the knees.

Patellar hypermobility, allowing the kneecap (patella) to move to one side of the leg, frequently to the lateral side (outside), is common in osteogenesis imperfecta. Ligament and tendon laxity, femoral bowing in the frontal plane, and muscular imbalance of the quadriceps muscles are potential contributors. It is not unusual for this to increase during a period of immobilization of the femur after a fracture or surgical procedure, suggesting muscular weakness or imbalance is contributory. Selective strengthening of the medial (inside) quadriceps and the adductor muscles on the inside of the leg can help realign the patella if the source of the problem is muscular. A knee cuff or sleeve can also be helpful for some children, particularly during walking.

Limited knee extension, in which the hamstring muscles that flex the knee and adjacent soft tissues become shortened, presents a significant challenge. It is essential to make an effort to analyze and identify potential sources of the shortening. Limited knee extension is usually not associated with femoral rod migration. More commonly this presents as limited, painful knee flexion (bending). However, poor femoral rod orientation above the knee can cause pain and reduce the ability to fully extend the knee. Once again, structural limitations, including tibial rod migration, should be ruled out as sources of limitation before beginning an intervention program to increase range of motion.

If it is determined that limited knee extension is of muscular and other soft tissue origin, the next step is to consider why the tissues have shortened. *Limited knee extension in only one knee joint* is common after fracture or surgery if the knee has been immobilized in flexion. This usually responds quickly to activities in the water emphasizing all hip motions, as well as knee flexion and extension. Activities out of the water focus on active end range extension (the last 30 degrees) in supine, prone, long sitting (knees fully extended), and in short sitting (knees flexed), with the leg supported. If range is not improving fairly quickly, the patella may be "bound down" and not tracking freely to allow smooth knee extension and flexion. The key is to first determine if this is the case, and second to recognize that too much patellar mobility creates other problems in osteogenesis imperfecta, such as lateral subluxation of the patella. Increasing patellar mobility gradually through gentle friction massage can help regain patellar movement in an up-and-down direction, needed for improved knee flexion and extension, while not increasing it in a lateral or sideways direction.

Using active movements to increase knee extension may appear conservative, but it is less likely to create other joint abnormalities. Putting a weight on top of the knee to make it straighter or using passive stretching methods may create other problems. In a system that is physiologically hyperflexible, passive stretching methods elongate the soft tissue components that offer the least resistance, often not the ones that are most responsible for movement limitation.

When both knees are tight in flexion, and therefore have limited knee extension, the limited extension can be transitional after immobilization in a spica cast, but it is more likely linked to long-term sitting, particularly if the hips are also limited in extension. The choices here are to spend a large amount of time and effort exercising to increase the knee and (usually) hip extension, or to identify and address the source of the limitation. A combination of exercises to increase range of motion, in addition to life style changes to spend more time in positions other than sitting, is usually the most effective approach over the long term.

We discussed above the drawbacks of many hours of sustained sitting with the knees and hips in flexion. The influence on range of motion is obvious. Unless the knees and hips are extended for part of the waking hours of the day, it is a losing battle to accomplish more extension. Multiple approaches exist to increase extension, from use of a reclining wheelchair for a child who is unable to transfer out of the chair, to lying in extension on the couch in the nurse's office, to exercising on a mat or carpet in prone position at school or at home, to standing or walking at least once and up to two or three times during each school day. Which activity is selected depends on child and family preferences, and on what is reasonable in a particular school environment. The physical therapist for that school and the child's personal care aide can help structure this so that it occurs on a daily basis with minimal or no impact on the child's academic schedule, lunch with friends, or recess. It's a difficult balancing act, but it is possible, sometimes using a study hall.

Hyperflexibility at the hips usually presents as significantly more lateral or external rotation (legs rolling outward) than medial or internal rotation. Bias toward rolling the legs outward (hip external rotation) is common in osteogenesis imperfecta, and the source of it is more complicated than soft tissue laxity. Body position, opportunity for standing, and femoral bowing are among the potential contributors. Most young babies have 90 degrees of hip external rotation (their legs open completely and easily into a frog leg position) and only about half as much internal rotation. With growth and experience, this ratio is modified. As the legs begin to come together, external rotation is reduced and internal rotation increases. The earliest steps in this process are evident as the supine baby is able to pull the widely spaced legs upward and together to kick against gravity. We discussed in Chapter 2 use of the buoyancy of water in the bathtub to assist infants with osteogenesis imperfecta with the process of pulling the legs up and together. Positioning in side-lying for infants and older children also helps to bring the legs together.

A similar process occurs in sitting. Early sitters have widely spaced legs to provide the broadest base of support for stability while sitting. Gradually they are able to maintain sitting with the knees closer together and fully extended (long sitting) or flexed over the edge of a sitting surface (short sitting). Infants and young children with osteogenesis imperfecta can benefit from early sitting with widely spaced knees to accomplish sitting. Recall, however, that we specifically emphasized in Chapter 2 that propped sitting with widely spaced legs should be avoided in order to promote development of an erect back. The same emphasis is appropriate in the present context. As soon as the child has achieved sitting with a wide base of support, it's time to move forward to develop a range of sitting skills with the legs closer together and to encourage active internal rotation and hip adduction (pulling the legs together) exercises.

Static leg position while sitting is also important. The sitter should be comfortable, and the ability to transfer smoothly into and out of a wheelchair is crucial. However, some children with widely spaced legs can benefit from lateral thigh supports on the wheelchair to encourage leg placement a little closer together. Since thigh supports can make transfers more difficult, it may be sufficient to make sure the foot plates are low enough to encourage straighter legs in the chair, rather than widely spaced legs resulting in weight-bearing on the outside of the knees. Straighter legs in the chair, combined with lateral thigh supports, can sometimes decrease spontaneous weight-shifting while sitting, potentially a source of back pain. Thus, the decision to use these or not depends on the needs, size, and abilities of each child.

Like sitting, standing also begins with a wide base of support and progresses in the same way, challenging the muscles that internally rotate the legs and pull them together beneath the pelvis. Children without standing experience frequently have widely spaced (abducted) and externally rotated legs. Children with osteogenesis imperfecta often revert to this pattern after a long period of non-weight-bearing associated with recovery from fracture or surgery. However, even very high-performing children with osteogenesis imperfecta may have far more external than internal hip rotation, suggesting that this is linked to factors beyond weakness, positioning, or ligamentous laxity.

Providing standing opportunities to attain or regain this skill, using devices as needed, helps to activate the muscles that pull the legs together. This is most effective in younger children. Recall that we discussed in Chapter 2 placing emphasis on learning to walk forward, with external support, for new walkers rather than encouraging a prolonged period of sidestepping or cruising. Established walkers with osteogenesis imperfecta often maintain a wide base of support, with externally rotated legs, as a result of hip muscle weakness rather than range of motion disparity. The ratio of external to internal rotation will not change in standing until weakness is identified and addressed. In addition to exercises to increase hip abduction and adduction strength on each side, straight leg raising in a diagonal pattern that links hip flexion, internal rotation, and adduction with knee extension can be helpful to improve the rotation ratio during standing and walking.

Hip range of motion limitation most often presents as the inability to gain full hip extension in any body position. It is most evident in standing, when the pelvis extends outward in back, and the child cannot pull the pelvis in and under the thorax, so that the legs are under the pelvis. This range of motion limitation has significant functional implications. It limits the size of the steps the child can take, how easily the leg can be lifted into the air to take steps, and gait efficiency in general. It often determines whether or not the child walks with an assistive device, and which one is most appropriate. Except for children 2 years of age or younger, who typically do not have full hip extension until their gait pattern has matured, limitations in hip extension are not helpful and should be addressed. The first place to start is to look at the child's amount of sustained sitting time during the day. Sustained sitting has to be interrupted in order to gain functional hip extension. The second is to analyze the pattern of muscle strength in the hips. If the hip flexors are much stronger than the hip extensors, which is often the case, exercises have to be devised to specifically strengthen the hip extensors, usually in conjunction with the knee extensors.

Although it is a common approach to strengthening hip extensors, *bridging (lifting the pelvis while backlying) may not be a good choice to strengthen hip and back extensor muscles in children with osteogenesis imperfecta*. Since bowing of the tibia is frequently in the sagittal plane in osteogenesis imperfecta, it might be prudent to avoid repetitive, high-challenge lifting of the hips, or bridging, in backlying while the knees are flexed with the feet planted. Of course, children need the capability to lift the pelvis in backlying as a life skill, but it is more effective to strengthen hip extensors with knee extension in prone, sit-to-standing, or standing to develop a linked extension pattern of stability.

In addition to active exercise to increase hip extension, positioning the body in trunk and hip extension for some portion of the day, lying in prone (Figure 3), standing or walking, supplemented by exercises, provide the advantage of active effort coupled with controlled soft tissue elongation. In contrast, passive manual stretching of hip flexors without interrupting sitting time to provide body extension is a burden for all concerned and has little potential for accomplishing effective change.

We've discussed above the most common patterns of limited or excessive joint mobility in children with osteogenesis imperfecta. Others that are less common but also require vigilance include hypermobility in the back, neck, elbow, thumb, and fingers. *Joint laxity and hypermobility in the back* may be one of several contributing factors to scoliosis. Given the triplanar mobility and complex relationships of the vertebral joints, it would be extremely difficult to devise activities to target and reduce the hypermobility. To date, exercise has not been demonstrated to be effective to reduce or stabilize scoliosis. However, strengthening the back muscles and associated connective tissues in straight plane activities, without rotation (twisting of the back), has functional utility and can be helpful with respect to alignment. There are many ways to do this, and appropriate choices have to be made for specific children. However, single arm (alternating) overhead reaching, which can be used to place some traction on the spine while at the same time recruiting the back muscles to elevate the arm, is a safe choice for most children. The abdominal muscles also influence trunk alignment and therefore the position of the back. Strengthening these muscles has clear functional benefit and can possibly influence alignment. Once again, choices of exercises are many, but given the risk of fracture with rotation, it's probably best to 1) concentrate on straight plane activities; 2) strengthen throughout the full arc of motion rather than just doing crunches; and 3) avoid lifting both straight legs simultaneously because of the stresses placed on the lower back.

Hypermobility in the neck can occur at the joint between the base of the skull (occiput) and the first bone (vertebra) of the spine. It frequently coexists with significantly large head size in proportion to the body. Sometimes there is a relative migration of the base of the skull downward over the cervical spine known as *basilar invagination*. This is typically identified and monitored with diagnostic imaging and may require ongoing consultation by a pediatric neurologist. Basilar invagination is asymptomatic in the majority of children, but when it is symptomatic, headaches are the most frequent problem. There is no evidence that hypermobility, large head size, or basilar invagination is related to physical activity. However, given the bone quality and joint hypermobility often associated with osteogenesis imperfecta, forward and backward somersaults should be avoided, except in the water. Gymnastics and diving from above the surface of the water should also be avoided.

Hyperflexibility at the elbow often takes the form of *subluxation of the head of the radius*, in which the forearm bone directly above the thumb slips outward at the elbow joint. Although the cause is joint laxity, the result is limitation in flexing the elbow, and sometimes rotating the forearm and the hand. This becomes a performance problem when the child cannot bring food to the mouth or turn doorknobs, or has difficulty brushing teeth or styling hair. Solving this problem requires surgical intervention. As radial head subluxation develops slowly, this can often be done at the same time as surgery for another purpose.

Thumb hyperflexibility, if present, usually occurs as hyperextension at the metacarpalphalangeal joint, located at the skin fold the thumb shares with the first finger. The primary impact of this is on strength in opposition, the ability to bring the thumb forcefully toward the fingers in order to grasp, hold, or pick up objects. Strengthening exercises to improve thumb flexion, adduction (thumb toward palm), and opposition may be helpful, but most of the time the problem is one of alignment rather than strength. A soft sleeve or a custom-made orthosis to stabilize the thumb may be necessary for improved function.

Similarly, **hyperflexibility in the fingers**, when present, is typically hyperextension. It may look like the fingers are double-jointed. Some of the extensor tendons may slip outside of the tracks in which they normally move, so that the finger "catches" at that joint, limiting end range movement. Many braces (orthoses) exist to stabilize these joints, ranging from off-the-shelf plastic devices to custom-fitted silver and gold rings. As the latter are beautiful (some can be ordered with gemstones) as well as effective, children rarely complain about having to wear them.

Strength and Weakness: Performance Emphasis for Middle Childhood

It follows from the discussion above that the balance of muscle strength across a joint, soft tissue hyper- or hypoflexibility, and alignment are related. Thus, one approach to improving joint mobility is through specific strengthening exercises for selected muscles. Similarly, exercises for specific muscle groups are often recommended in order to anticipate, or in response to, alignment problems related to osteogenesis imperfecta. In addition to these relationships, we know well that performance capabilities of children with osteogenesis imperfecta are broad, ranging from the ability to walk or run without adaptive devices to the need for powered locomotion. Finally, performance can be highly variable within the same child, who could walk easily before surgery for scoliosis, but cannot roll without assistance for some time afterward. Given this range of variation, general exercise recommendations for osteogenesis imperfecta are rarely appropriate. They must be based on the needs of each child.

In Chapter 2, considerable emphasis was placed on developing positive associations with movement and physical effort for infants and young children, rather than programming them beyond their ability to enjoy the activity or to cooperate. A similar approach can be effective with children in elementary and middle school if caregivers pay attention to what is important to the child, as well as the family, and look for ways to integrate activities into the child's day without making a burden for everyone.

In general, patterns of weakness influencing function are most often noted in the trunk and legs for children in elementary and middle school. Hypermobility in the hands and elbows, bowing in the upper or lower arm, or recent arm fracture can make upper extremity (arm) activities more difficult, but arm weakness is not typically a long-term limitation in this age group. In contrast, weakness in the trunk and legs, especially the hips, is common. Since any exercise program has to take into account joint alignment, or malalignment, as well as weakness, it is not a simple matter of "do this." Rather, it makes sense, for this age group, to approach it from the standpoint of the functional limitations related to weakness, and accomplishment of basic life skills leading to independence. For example, if the child cannot roll, the key is to analyze the pattern of weakness limiting the ability to complete this task, then address the weakness or alignment problem. Intended for any child with osteogenesis imperfecta, the same approach can be applied to accomplish all of the following BASIC COMPETENCIES.

*1) **Rolling in all directions:*** An essential competency, rolling is also an excellent exercise to extend the body and strengthen the trunk. If 20 to 25 repetitions or more are completed in each direction, it also becomes a good method to improve cardiorespiratory endurance for children who do not walk and spend a lot of time sitting.

*2) **Ability to lie prone for at least 5 minutes and up to 30 minutes:*** This requires the same skills to achieve it as rolling, so the inability to do so should be analyzed in a similar fashion. While in prone position, it may be worthwhile to try some mini-push-ups, hands flat, straightening the elbows only a few degrees, or an inch or so. If this goes well over several weeks or months, the child can push up to hands-and-knees position and ease down again for four to five comfortable repetitions. You may be surprised to find that some children with osteogenesis imperfecta can do actual push-ups with elbows and knees completely straight. If so, suggest not more than 10 to 15 at a time.

*3) **Ability to scoot or demonstrate some form of locomotion while prone, supine, or sitting:*** Scooting in supine is the most primitive among these types of locomotion, and it is an essential skill for individuals with osteogenesis imperfecta in order to move in a spica, or even a long leg cast. However, locomotor competence while prone and sitting are far more important life skills. At minimum, prone locomotion is the capability to scoot sideways, as if rotating around an umbilical axis, with the abdomen flat against the support surface. Inability to do this often relates to arm, hip, and trunk weakness, requiring analysis of weakness patterns for a particular child to determine how to achieve this skill. The ability to crawl on hands and knees is useful, but it is not an essential life skill. Spending many months to achieve this capability in young children with osteogenesis imperfecta reinforces hip and knee flexor dominance, and may not be the best use of time and resources. In contrast, the ability to scoot in sitting is the keystone for doing transfers among different body positions, including into and out of the wheelchair, and from sitting to standing.

If an elementary or middle school child cannot scoot in sitting, the first place to check is whether the hamstring muscles and tendons on the back of the thigh are tight, making it difficult to extend one leg forward at a time in order to move in sitting. Wearing slippery shorts or pants often solves this problem in the short term. But efforts to elongate the hamstrings through long sitting positioning, and increased out-of-chair time with the knees in extension can solve this problem over the long term. More commonly a child who could scoot before an arm fracture loses the ability to do so. If the abdominal muscles have sufficient strength, it is relatively easy to teach this child to tilt the body to one side in order to unload and advance the opposite leg, then repeat the pattern on the other side. Scooting then becomes possible using only the legs, an incredibly liberating way to move.

4) Ability to sit up from supine: This is a skill most people take for granted, but it can be a difficult challenge for children with osteogenesis imperfecta. Not simply a matter of abdominal muscle strength, the ability to sit up also depends on the strength of the muscles that stabilize the legs and bend the trunk, and the relative proportions of trunk length and leg length. Sitting up is especially difficult for children with short legs in relation to the length of the trunk. Despite this, sitting up independently, perhaps using the arms, is a reasonable expectation for the majority of children with osteogenesis imperfecta (an important exception is following recent back or hip surgery). Children who cannot sit straight up because of back surgery or weakness generally turn to the side and push up with one or both arms. For a child who cannot sit up at all because of weakness or recent fracture, this is the recommended method to begin to teach this skill. Once this is under way, emphasis shifts to strengthening the abdominal and hip flexor muscles that flex the trunk in relation to the legs.

It is important to include the entire arc of movement from lying flat to sitting up straight. Working only on crunches, the current trend, challenges the

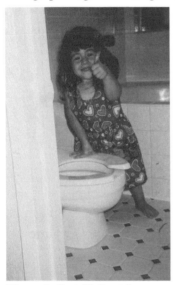

muscles at only one end of the functional arc of movement. A more comprehensive approach is to work from both ends of the arc and try to meet in the middle. The top of the arc is addressed by doing sit-ups from a fairly high support surface so the child is close to vertical when beginning the sit-up, and succeeds in doing this independently. Very gradually, over the course of weeks or months, the pillow support or wedge is lowered as the child continues to succeed while getting stronger and more capable functionally. If this is done gradually, without the sense of an enormous amount of effort, children frequently challenge themselves to do more, and delight in the accomplishment. Straight plane arcs, rather than rotation (shoulder toward the opposite knee) are usually preferred because

Figure 5. Installation of a pedi toilet can be the means to achieve full independence at home.

of the increased fracture risk with rotation (twisting) throughout the body.

5) Independent dressing and toileting, and minimal assistance for bathing: Independent dressing should be possible even for a child who cannot sit, but can roll. Creative clothing selection solves most problems; for instance, neck openings that are not too tight, pants of flexible rather than rigid material, Velcro shoe closures or elastic laces if getting shoes on and off is a problem. Limitations to independent toileting can include weakness, especially in the arms and trunk, or inaccessibility of the wheelchair to the toilet. Resolving this depends on identifying the constraints in a particular situation (Figure 5). It may be as basic as putting an inexpensive insert inside the toilet seat at school so the opening is smaller and the child feels more secure. For children who cannot stand, a hi-low power chair may be necessary to achieve independent toileting. A similar approach to bathing should focus on the long-term goal of complete independence using a shower or bathtub and adaptive devices as needed. Many exist to accomplish this; they are described in Chapter 7.

6) Ability to transfer into and out of all body positions independently, except standing, using assistive devices as needed: It may be difficult for parents to break the habit of "parent pick-up and place" that develops quite naturally when children with osteogenesis imperfecta are younger or in pain. Since it is often much faster than waiting for the child to move into and out of various positions, this easily becomes an established behavior. The difficulty with this approach is that children will outgrow their parents' ability to lift their weight to place them. Thus, it is clearly an advantage to encourage independent transfers by young children, and to expect them from children in school.

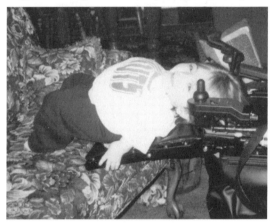

Figure 6. Use of a specialized power chair for independent transfer from wheelchair to sofa for a child who transfers in backlying position.

This may require creative thinking in the short term for children who have had a fracture recently and may need to be manually lifted until the fracture heals. For children who are unable to carry out independent transfers over the long term because of weakness, especially in the arms and trunk, or fracture nonunion, or obesity, a vast array of adaptive devices exists to make this possible (Figure 6). For example, a hi-low power chair can provide complete or almost complete independence for a child who otherwise would have to be constantly lifted. However, use of a power chair requires the means to transport a heavy device with a large footprint, and the environmental access to be able to use it to the child's full potential. This approach and many others are described in detail in Chapter 7.

7) Daily standing for 30 to 60 minutes with a supine stander, or walking: Finding a balance in one's day between activity and sitting is a challenge for each of us. Obesity, back pain, tight muscles, and poor cardiorespiratory endurance are indicators that the body is out of balance. This becomes particularly challenging for non-walking children with osteogenesis imperfecta who are approaching adolescence. Many recreational activities are appropriate and satisfying for children in chairs, but getting out of the chair and using a standing device once or twice a day for 30 minutes is a significant step toward maintaining the balance of flexion and extension for one's body. A supine or upright stander also can be useful for walking children who have had an arm fracture, or as a means of transition to re-establish walking after a prolonged period of convalescence (Figure 7). How much emphasis to place on walking is a decision made by the parents and the child with osteogenesis imperfecta. However, daily effort focused on standing provides many benefits, not the least of which is the ability to take at least partial responsibility for one's own body weight in standing.

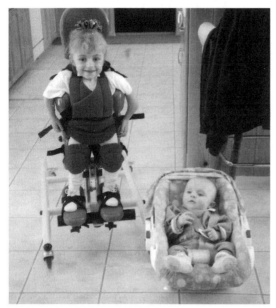

Figure 7. Use of a supine stander, when walking is not possible.

8) Singing, playing a musical instrument, or other cardiopulmonary activity: In the same way that muscles move the legs and arms, the power source for the chest is muscular. For individuals who are quite active, the chest to a large extent takes care of itself; that is, the deep breathing necessary to support body activities, especially recreational ones, provides the challenge to attain muscular efficiency and increase lung capacity. Children with osteogenesis imperfecta have two issues to face: the first is that bones, muscles, and the connective tissues of the chest wall can grow in a creative manner, producing chest impairments such as pectus carinatum or pectus excavatum. The second is that lack of body activity over the long term because of weakness, fractures, or obesity does not provide sufficient challenge for the development of muscular efficiency and lung capacity. The good news is that the cardiorespiratory system, especially lung capacity, continues to develop into the early twenties, so ample time exists to improve lung capacity and muscular efficiency.

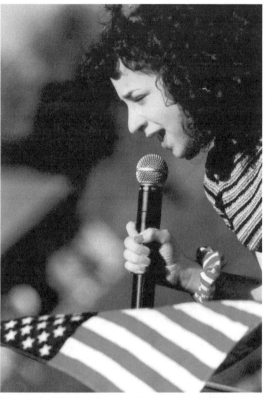

Figure 8. Singing is a good choice for building pulmonary capacity and endurance.

The key, however, is how to do this. What is appropriate for a specific child? The first intervention is simply to remember that the chest also needs exercise challenge. The second is to consider the range of possibilities and work with the child to select something that can be done consistently. Children who cannot transfer into and out of sitting can achieve exertional activity through rolling repetitions, an example already described above. But singing in the chorus, taking voice lessons, playing a recorder or other wind instrument, or swimming three to four times a week will specifically develop cardiopulmonary endurance and capacity. Although not as essential, the same or similar activities should also be considered for children who are walking most of the day. Recall that as children get older, they spend increasing time in sitting during the school day and doing homework after school. This happens so gradually that most of us aren't really aware of it. With the knowledge that this is inevitable, it becomes increasing-

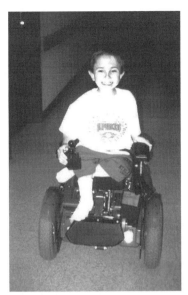

Figure 9. Achieving independence in various domains of function, including recreation, with use of a hi-low power chair.

ly important for parents and their children with osteogenesis imperfecta to secure some time during the day for activities that require very deep breaths and elevate the heart rate (Figure 8).

9) Recreational activities: Pursuit of one or more recreational interests is beneficial in many respects for everyone. Numerous recreational opportunities are possible for children with osteogenesis imperfecta, and many are described in Chapter 6. Middle childhood is the logical time for children and parents to begin the transition from consistent reliance on therapy-guided exercise programs toward supplemental recreational activities that integrate the child socially (Figure 9). As children get older, it becomes increasingly difficult to do straight plane exercises at school, or to stand on the supine stander, and still accomplish everything else that has to be done there. Thus, the emphasis shifts to identifying what the child cannot manage at school, for instance, independent toileting, and working with the therapy team to determine how to accomplish a specific objective like this one. This is often synchronous with a gradual shift from direct therapy toward adaptive physical education, and eventually, the child may be fully integrated into the same physical education class as his or her age mates. The way in which this process occurs will differ substantially depending on the interests and performance level of the child, the parents' priorities, and the general tenor of the school and the school district.

Anticipating Adolescence

Many ideas have been discussed in this chapter in an effort to be as inclusive as possible. Naturally, all of the recommendations are not applicable to all children with osteogenesis imperfecta. Parents and their children need the freedom to make their own choices, and not be burdened by alternatives that are not appropriate for their child or their family. In anticipation of adolescence, we conclude this chapter by encouraging parents to remember that the first rule of childhood is to have fun, and to balance the work day so that some fun is possible. A second consideration as high school becomes imminent is to ask, "How are we doing?" As basic as this sounds, it can help parents and children focus on what they have accomplished so far, and what performance objective they want to focus on next. Finally, parents should anticipate that the transition to adolescence may be challenging, as children make discoveries about who they are, and parents learn to let them.

Summary points:

- Middle childhood is the interval of opportunity to promote the transition from the dependence of early childhood to the independence of adolescence.

- To the extent possible, expectations for children should nurture their sense of self-competence, rather than place them in the position of constantly trying to please adults.

- Focusing on accomplishing one performance objective at a time is often more effective than fragmented efforts in multiple areas.

- Relationships among strength, alignment, and joint range of motion are complex, requiring careful analysis of their interplay in order to target interventions precisely.

- Early indications of obesity or limited range of motion in the hips and knees merit a close look at the amount of time the child spends sitting in the wheelchair.

- Increasing activity levels, and the development of cardiorespiratory capacity through recreational opportunities, has lifelong benefits in addition to being a lot of fun.

- Passive stretching of short muscles is rarely effective and may lead to undesirable joint laxity unless the reason they are short is identified and remediated.

- Daily opportunities to stand, walk, or lie in prone with the hips and knees extended are critical to maintain the ability to extend the legs.

- Having fun is a top priority for all children. If exercise is too burdensome, it's time to re-evaluate.

CHAPTER FOUR

STRATEGIES FOR ADOLESCENTS

Transitional approaches to promote independence

Scott M. Paul, MD

Goals for adolescence, the transition to independent adulthood:
- Understand, as parents and caregivers, the physical and psychological issues of adolescence in general and for people with osteogenesis imperfecta in order to support the adolescent's successful transition to adulthood
- Encourage adolescents to gradually make a successful transition from partnering with parents to taking full responsibility for independent function in all domains of life, including their health and rehabilitation programs
- Help the adolescent learn how to cope with the demands and pleasures associated with independent adulthood

Charting the Course to Adulthood: Is Independence the Goal?

After the period of gradual growth and acquisition of skills that is associated with the "wonder years" of childhood, changes become more precipitous around the time girls approach 11 or 12 years and boys approach 12 or 13 years of age. Adolescence is the time of transition from the dependence of childhood to the independence of adulthood. Hormones begin to signal the body to launch the process toward adulthood.

During adolescence, these "pre-adults" need to take increasing control of their lives. Parents have to guide their child's explorations into increased control in such a way that social and behavioral development is in synchrony with physical growth and development (Table 1). The parents of adolescents with osteogenesis imperfecta also have to contend with guiding these explorations

Table 1. Normal Developmental Progress in Adolescence.

Sphere of Development	Early Adolescence	Middle Adolescence	Late Adolescence
Social	Close friendships gain importance Peer group influences interests and clothing styles	Effort to make new friends Strong emphasis on new peer group and group identity of selectivity, superiority, and competitiveness	Ability to compromise Self-reliance Greater concern for others
Emotional	Moodiness Less attention shown to parents, with occasional rudeness Tendency to return to childish behavior, fought off by excessive activity Rule and limit testing Occasional experimenting with cigarettes, marijuana, and alcohol	Self-involvement, alternating between unrealistically high expectations and poor self-concept Complaints that parents interfere with independence Extremely concerned with appearance and one's own body Feelings of strangeness about oneself and one's body Lowered opinion of parents, withdrawal of emotions from them Periods of sadness as psychological loss of parents takes place	Firmer identity Ability to delay gratification More developed sense of humor Greater emotional stability Stable interests Pride in one's work
Intellectual	Struggle with sense of identity Capacity for abstract thought Improved ability to use speech to express oneself, but more likely to express feelings by actions than by words	Close to full achievement of adult verbal skills, still developing written skills Examination of inner experiences, which may include maintaining a diary	Ability to think ideas through Ability to make independent decisions Ability to express ideas in words, full achievement of adult verbal skills, close to full achievement of adult written skills
Physical	Further increases in body strength, with beginnings of adult muscle development	Close to full achievement of individual's adult strength and skills	Full achievement of individual's adult strength and skills

Table 1. Normal Developmental Progress in Adolescence (continued).

Sphere of Development	Early Adolescence	Middle Adolescence	Late Adolescence
Sexual	Pubic hair develops	Pubic hair fills in	Adult sexual charac- teristics (although some
	Scrotum begins to enlarge in boys	Breast enlargement in girls	boys may not com- plete maturation until 21 or 22 years old)
	Breast development begins in girls	Penis enlarges and further scrotal enlarge- ment in boys	
	Many girls reach menarche by age 14		

in a situation where social and behavioral development is not necessarily synchronous with normative physical growth and development. The 7 to 10 years of this transition are a challenge for any adolescent and his or her family (see also Chapters 2 and 3 on preadolescent development).

Neither children nor adults, adolescents must live and learn to cope with the awkwardness of this transitional state. The process can be eased by the support and understanding of their parents. As part of the learning process, adolescents frequently take risks and challenge authority. The adolescent's parents and caregivers must walk a tightrope between granting privileges and placing limits on the adolescent's activities. The dilemma facing parents and caregivers of adolescents who have osteogenesis imperfecta is amplified by concerns about the risk of fractures with increased activity on the one hand, and the risks associated with inactivity and obesity resulting from poor compliance with exercise and healthy behaviors on the other. This chapter offers suggestions that may be helpful to facilitate as smooth a journey through adolescence as possible.

Turn and Face the Strange Changes

As with any other child, childhood for youngsters with osteogenesis imperfecta has been a time when they have learned much about their personal strengths and challenges. They should already have some good insights into the nature of their impairments and how to cope with the functional problems created by those impairments. Their parents should have a good understanding of the impairments and disabilities that have affected their child's life and the interventions that have helped to reduce impairment and improve function.

The first step on the road to successful adulthood is for parents to help the adolescent with osteogenesis imperfecta remember the lessons already learned and to build on this knowledge. The next step is appreciating and understanding the changes that occur in the adolescent's body. These changes can be very sudden and precipitous. An awareness of these changes before they occur allows the family to react more quickly and develop successful strategies to manage the changes.

Growth in Height and Weight

Hormones typically signal rapid changes in height and body proportions during adolescence. Height will probably not change as much in many adolescents with osteogenesis imperfecta because of the underlying problems with collagen, previous fractures, and problems with the plates of cells at either end of the bones where growth occurs. However, any growth changes the position of the body's center of gravity. The change in center of gravity affects balance in sitting, standing, and walking. In addition, growth on one side of the body in osteogenesis imperfecta can be more rapid or greater than on the other, which also affects the balance of the adolescent when sitting, standing, or walking. These changes increase the risk of falls or may change the ability to walk. Growth imbalance can also put increased stresses on the spine if not corrected.

Along with growth in height, the hormones also signal breast development in girls, new fat distributions (more in girls than in boys), and the addition of muscle mass in both girls and boys. In addition to body image issues (see below), these changes can also affect balance in sitting, standing, and walking. This is the period when the risk of weight gain and loss of ability to walk is greatest. Changes in both length and body proportions can also affect bed mobility and ability to transfer into and out of bed.

Strategies to manage growth changes:
- Exercises to increase back, abdominal, and limb strength, promote symmetrical, flexible range of motion in joints, and increase balance can help address these issues.
- Shoe lifts to level leg length can be useful for some adolescents.

- Walking assistance devices, such as walkers or crutches, should be modified to accommodate for growth.
- If there are spine deformities for which surgical correction has been considered, it is appropriate to ask if growth is sufficiently completed before undergoing spine surgery.

Sexual Maturation

The same hormones that start the rapid changes in growth and body appearance also begin the process of sexual maturation. Body hair begins to transform to adult patterns of growth and the sexual organs mature. Although osteogenesis imperfecta can delay sexual maturity, it does not prevent puberty or fertility. This means that girls with osteogenesis imperfecta may be physically able to become pregnant at or before age 14 or 15 years and boys with osteogenesis imperfecta may be able to successfully impregnate a sexual partner at or before age 15 or 16 years.

In society, however, there is a tendency for some people with disabilities to be viewed as asexual. *This is not accurate* from either a physiological or an emotional standpoint. It is important for families to consider how and what they will teach their adolescents with osteogenesis imperfecta in terms of sex education. To avoid the subject is to risk the adolescent's learning through misinformation and allowing the philosophy of the prevailing teen culture to be adopted, rather than the family's mores and beliefs. This issue can be even more important for the adolescent with osteogenesis imperfecta, because of the potential complications related to sexual intercourse and pregnancy that an adolescent or adult with osteogenesis imperfecta faces.

Strategies to cope with emerging sexuality:
- Parents should agree on their philosophy toward dating and sexual activity before the child reaches adolescence.
- Parents need to share their beliefs with their child with osteogenesis imperfecta before the child is likely to encounter external pressures from television, movies, and peers.
- When adolescents are seriously considering becoming sexually active, they should be encouraged to speak with their physicians and therapists about how osteogenesis imperfecta, their specific disabilities, and the risk of

injury may require them to adapt the mechanics of sexual intercourse, and how pregnancy can affect their bodies.

Social Maturity and Integration

Great emotional challenges are involved in coping with these momentous changes. They are made more complicated by the very hormones that are causing these changes, which can also cause frequent and wide mood swings. Most adolescents struggle with being "different" and not being "popular." Having osteogenesis imperfecta may amplify these feelings. Adolescents are coming to terms with their own image of themselves and are judging themselves by how they are viewed by peers. There is a desire to be part of a group. Social norms are learned by interactions within these groups. Group activities pro-

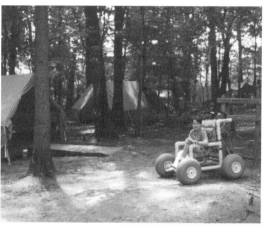

Figure 1. Using an all-terrain wheelchair to make camping with the Boy Scouts possible for an adolescent with osteogenesis imperfecta.

vide opportunities for adolescents to experiment with making decisions independently of their parents. The limitations in mobility faced by many adolescents with osteogenesis imperfecta may place obstacles in front of some activities. Despite this, parents should encourage adolescents to participate in low-risk recreational activities with their peers in order to help them develop a sense of accomplishment and acceptance.

Since the adoption of the Americans with Disabilities Act, schools, churches, and organized community groups such as the Scouts have become more sensitive to the needs of people with disabilities. Adolescents (and their families) should be encouraged to help educate leaders in these groups about the specific abilities and challenges they face, in order to promote participation in activities that interest them. Adolescents, as well as their parents, should be willing to enlist their healthcare and rehabilitation teams to assist with this educational process. (Figure 1 shows how one family solved the challenge of participating in camping activities.) This process of educating the people involved is, in itself, an important experience for adolescents, since they will be faced with similar situations at work and other social environments as adults.

Parents of children with osteogenesis imperfecta actually have some advantages over parents of nondisabled adolescents. They have already learned how to emotionally support a child who feels different from others. They have had to find the balance of promoting independence while protecting their child from harm. Assisting an adolescent's growth into an adult is more of the same. The difference in adolescence is that more patience will be required of parents while providing emotional support because of the mood and image challenges discussed above, especially now that the balance between protection and independence needs to tip in favor of promoting independence.

Similarly, adolescents with osteogenesis imperfecta should be encouraged to understand that they have already successfully met some of the challenges their peers are facing only now. Adolescents with osteogenesis imperfecta have already learned more about their emotional and physical strengths and weaknesses than the average able-bodied adolescent.

Strategies for social growth:
- Encourage involvement in organized youth groups that include nondisabled and disabled adolescents.
- Schedule visits with the adolescent's medical and rehabilitation teams to work out adaptations required to maintain participation in social activities.
- Provide opportunities for the adolescent to discuss his or her social life without the parents seeming to pry.
- Seek professional support from a social worker or psychologist if there are serious concerns.
- Consider planning for the ability to drive, which can help promote the adolescent's social integration.

Learning to Pilot the Ship: Taking Charge of Change
To grow into successful adults, adolescents with osteogenesis imperfecta must do more than just understand the changes they and their peers are experienc-

ing. Adolescents with osteogenesis imperfecta should not just let changes happen; they should take charge of change!

Adolescents should actively strive to build a better body, mind, and soul. They need to use their knowledge of the course of change and apply it to forming regular good habits that will ease their transition and make them more successful as adults. Adolescents also need to know that failing to take responsibility for developing good health and exercise habits can lead to increased difficulties in even maintaining their current level of activity and function (Table 2). Just as good health and activity will increase their ability to function, lack of activity and poor health choices will push them down a slippery slope of increasing disability.

Building Your Best Body

The first step toward the best possible function in adulthood is to build a body that can support the capabilities needed to do required and desirable activities. This requires the best possible physical condition that the body will allow. Although there are many aspects to building a better body for adulthood, one crucial area for many adolescents with osteogenesis imperfecta (especially those whose mobility is limited) is the challenge of unhealthy weight gain and obesity. Maintaining a healthy body weight is a serious challenge.

Obesity is reaching epidemic proportions in the general population of the United States. It has increased the incidence of chronic illnesses such as diabetes and osteoarthritis (two diseases that can have devastating effects in adults with osteogenesis imperfecta) as well as heart disease. Abnormalities in body proportion and metabolism in adolescence can increase the risk of becoming overweight in some instances. This makes adolescents with osteogenesis imperfecta at very high risk for obesity.

Although the risk of arthritis should be warning enough for someone with a bone disorder like osteogenesis imperfecta, there are also risks of isolation from peer groups if significant weight gain limits social opportunities and physical participation. Controlling weight is a challenge for many and a greater challenge for those with osteogenesis imperfecta, whose disabilities may limit their activities. Obesity can become a vicious cycle for adolescents with osteogenesis imperfecta. It is harder to move larger bodies that have a higher center of gravity. As the weight increases, it becomes even harder. This can lead to decreased activity. Decreased activity leads to further weight gain.

Table 2. Some Risks of Not Responding to Change.

Change Taking Place	Risk	Suggestions to Reduce Risk
Increase in body fat	Excessive weight gain and loss of mobility Distortion of body image and shape	Less fast food, more healthy snacks; participation in exercise, sports, and family chores to adolescent's ability level; family reinforcement of health-supporting behaviors
Growth in height and change in body proportions	Increased effort to walk and resultant decreased desire to walk	Incentives to want to continue walking, such as fashionable (but properly fitting) shoes and sporty designs on orthotics
Increased socialization with peers without adult supervision	Alcohol or drug use with higher risks than in adolescents without osteogenesis imperfecta because of injury risk while impaired	Proactive discussion by parents about drug and alcohol risks in early adolescence; parents also need to maintain regular interest in adolescent's schedule and know adolescent's friends
Sexual maturity	Unanticipated pregnancy; sexually transmitted diseases; emotional scarring	Open discussions between parents and adolescent

This leads to a further decrease in activity. And so it goes.

Adolescents with osteogenesis imperfecta need to understand that there are only two ways to lose weight. Either you limit the calories going in or you burn more calories through increased activity. To help control appetite and limit the calories going in, adolescents should eat a healthy breakfast to start the day. They should consider packing a healthy lunch for school instead of buying fast food, high in fat and carbohydrates. If they note that clothing is getting tight or that it is getting harder to transfer, they should be aware that those are warning signs of weight gain. If they are having difficulty controlling their diet, they should seek the help and support of a registered dietitian who has had experience with adolescents with mobility impairments. Adolescents should also remember that the most pleasurable way to lose and keep off weight is to increase their physical activity as much as possible (as discussed in Chapters 2, 3, 5, and 6, and the paragraphs below).

Strength and flexibility are important not only for mobility and self-care, but also for good heart and lung function. One of the most important areas of the body to keep strong for comfortable sitting and good breathing is the trunk muscles. Many people with osteogenesis imperfecta have curves in the spine and/or deformities of the ribs. Exercise may or may not be able to change these deformities, but it will certainly slow or stop the progression of these problems. Adolescents should work with their rehabilitation physician and physical therapist to develop an exercise program that will maintain good flexibility of the spine and strengthen the abdominal and back muscles. Overhead arm reaching exercises can help stretch out the spine and rib cage. Adolescents should also ask their rehabilitation team about exercises that directly strengthen the breathing muscles of the diaphragm and ribs to improve lung capacity if they are unable to participate in recreational activities that provide this. Although back braces are often used to help support the spine, they should be used with caution in osteogenesis imperfecta for reasons including the "softness" of the bones resulting in a risk of further deformity being caused by the brace. Braces also result in weaker back and abdominal muscles because the brace takes over the work of the muscles, limiting the muscles' opportunity to exercise.

The strength of the legs should not be neglected in adolescence. For children with osteogenesis imperfecta who are able to walk, some strength will simply come from walking around. However, because of the deformities in spine and leg bones, the process of walking may not work muscles and joints evenly. Therefore, walking adolescents should still meet with their rehabilitation team to develop and adjust a regular exercise program to keep the legs strong and limber.

For adolescents who are unable to walk functionally, it is still valuable for them to ask their rehabilitation team about the development of exercises and use of equipment to try to achieve standing. As mentioned above, adolescents are growing to their adult height and weight. With growth, it becomes more difficult to rely on other people to transfer to the wheelchair, to the toilet, or to the tub. Therefore, it is very important for adolescents to develop and maintain the ability to stand and transfer, if at all possible. Otherwise, they may have to rely on home attendant services for help, which can be difficult to obtain and will limit their independence as adults in college, at work, and while traveling.

The health of the heart is related to the type of exercise called aerobics, which includes running, bicycling, swimming, and many sports. Although some of these activities may not be possible for some adolescents with osteogenesis imperfecta, they should be encouraged to find a sport or activity that they can enjoy doing regularly. Swimming is an especially good way to get aerobic, flexibility, and strength exercise in a safe setting. Aerobic exercise is important not only for the heart. Physical inactivity and the "American" diet, high in fat and carbohydrates, are serious risk factors for the development of obesity. Aerobic exercise not only helps the adolescent with osteogenesis imperfecta develop heart-healthy adult behaviors, but also reduces the risk of becoming overweight.

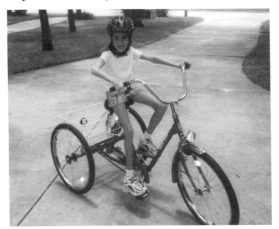

Figure 2: Many options exist for fun and aerobic exercise for adolescents with osteogenesis imperfecta.

Adolescents who are involved in exercise will gain self-esteem from seeing improvement over time and in mastering a challenging skill. The improved body image that comes from keeping weight under control will also help with self-esteem. Therefore, adolescents with osteogenesis imperfecta who are unable to participate in the sport of their choice in a standard way should know that many sports have been adapted for people with disabilities (see Chapter 6). Figure 2 shows how one adolescent was able to make adaptations in order to cycle. Adolescents might be encouraged to watch disabled sports events such as the Paralympics Games to see how people with disabilities participate in sports even at an elite level. To learn about opportunities for participation in sports for people with disabilities, adolescents and their families should be encouraged to contact their local rehabilitation hospital, county parks and recreation department, or national sports-with-disabilities organizations such as Disabled Sports USA and Wheelchair Sports USA (see Chapters 6 and 8).

Some adolescents with osteogenesis imperfecta have weakness, bowing, contractures, or joint problems in their arms, wrists, or hands. These can limit self-care activities such as washing and dressing. Even if self-care is not impaired, these deficits can cause difficulties with important activities of daily living such as cooking, writing, using a keyboard, or driving. Therefore, adolescents should still meet with their rehabilitation team, including the occupational therapist, to develop and adjust a regular exercise program to keep the arms as strong and limber as possible. The occupational therapist can also identify strategies to help with the independent performance of activities of daily living, including the use of adaptive equipment such as sock aids and button hookers.

Visits to medical professionals have, of necessity, been integrated into the daily lives of families of children with osteogenesis imperfecta. Because of this, families can become acclimated to maintaining very close contact with medical professionals, including physicians, nurses, physical therapists, and occupational therapists. By adolescence, healthy behaviors and a regular rehabilitation regimen should be well understood and routine. Since this is a time of growth into independence, adolescents with osteogenesis imperfecta and their families should be developing the ability to identify the times when help from their medical and rehabilitation teams is needed and distinguish them from the times when they can solve problems independently.

Although adolescence is the time to learn to take responsibility for oneself, adolescents with osteogenesis imperfecta need to know when to ask for help. Adolescents with more than a mild cold or other illness should still see their physician. When injuries occur, if there is significant pain and possibly a fracture, they should seek help. It is valuable to guide the adolescent into assuming the role of decision maker with the medical and rehabilitation teams, which can include learning to speak directly with health professionals, scheduling and keeping appointments, and renewing prescriptions. In some instances, this could also include parents stepping out of the room during medical history taking, physical examinations, and treatment sessions.

Taking It on the Road

Part of independence is being able to get around on your own and the many human-powered ways of getting around can also be good exercise. As in many activities, adolescents need to balance the health and fun benefits of wheeled activities, such as riding cycles and scooters, with the risk of falls and fractures. If, in close consultation with the doctor and therapists, adolescents and their parents agree that a wheeled activity is a risk worth taking, the adolescent should start slowly. Level, smooth, uncrowded areas should be chosen when the activity is first tried. It is important to wear proper safety gear during these activities to reduce the risk of injury. A certified helmet must be worn during any of these activities. The helmet must be fit properly when purchased and be worn so that it covers the forehead and protects the brain (see Chapter 6). It is also wise to wear elbow and arm pads. When using roller blades, skateboards, or scooters, it is important to wear a helmet, elbow and knee pads, and gloves. The adolescent should not do the activity alone. As skills improve, more difficult techniques can be considered.

For adolescents whose physical limitations do not permit these activities or where the risk of fractures would be too great, there are other human-powered activities they can participate in (see Chapter 6). Placing training wheels on a bicycle to stabilize it can be appropriate for some adolescents. For others, a full-size three-wheeled bicycle can provide sufficient stability while offering independence on wheels.

Taking It on the Road: Driving

The most important kind of wheeled mobility for most adolescents is the car. Learning to drive is a very important milestone that wraps within it many of the issues of adolescence, including increasing control, risk-taking behaviors, and coping with peer pressure. For these reasons, many states have instituted a "rookie driver" graduated license system. Whether or not your state has such a system, while planning for driving, it is important for adolescents and their parents to talk about these issues and revisit them as the time to begin driving approaches. Many adolescents will need special adaptations to drive. These adaptations can include pedal extensions, seat adaptations, and hand controls. Most school driver's education programs are not able to directly accommodate these needs, but each state has an office that addresses the vocational needs of people with disabilities. This state office will have a name such as Bureau of Vocational Rehabilitation or Department of Rehabilitation Services.

The family of an adolescent with osteogenesis imperfecta should meet with the rehabilitation team to help them decide when driver's education is appropriate for the adolescent and how to determine what adaptations will likely be necessary. The family should then contact resources such as the state office that provides vocational rehabilitation, the rehabilitation technology office of the school district, or a local rehabilitation hospital in order to locate a driving program for people with disabilities. The parents should visit prospective schools to ensure that they have the ability to assess the driving adaptation needs of the adolescent and provide an automobile with the accommodations required for the adolescent to appropriately learn to drive. When the time comes to adapt a car for the adolescent's needs, the family should speak with the state office that provides vocational rehabilitation, since financial assistance may be available to make the modifications. Most major automakers also have programs to help defray some costs of adaptations.

Building Who You Are

Adolescents who are successfully managing their health and physical condition have achieved a great deal. However, that is only the beginning. If adolescence is the transition to adulthood, it must be the time for adolescents to begin to think about the adult they'd like to be. It is a time when ideals, mores, and beliefs will be tested and accepted or rejected. It is the time when the adult "self" begins to form. Unfortunately, this self does not form in a vacuum. The self is judged against peers. Self usually begins with self-doubt and only later does self-confidence form.

Strategies for building a confident self-image:
• The family and the adolescent with osteogenesis imperfecta should not try to ignore the self-image challenges related to physical appearance. Neither should they overemphasize them. Figure 3 shows how one teen with osteogenesis imperfecta radiates a confident self-image that neither emphasizes nor deemphasizes her disabilities.
• The concept of "differently able" rather than disabled can be an effective guiding principle for coping with self-image issues related to osteogenesis imperfecta.
• One effective way to help adolescents is to find successful adults with osteogenesis imperfecta who can serve as peer supports by sharing their experiences.
• Adolescents should feel comfortable about seeking professional counseling if needed and should view this not as a weakness on their part, but as a strength of insight.

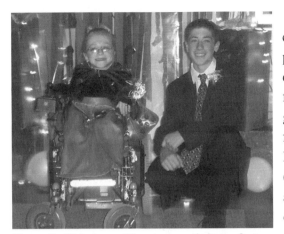

Figure 3: This teen with osteogenesis imperfecta is dressed to the nines and radiates a confident self-image at the Homecoming Dance.

Well-adjusted adolescents with osteogenesis imperfecta still need to consider issues related to their future. What are their career goals? Can their chosen profession be performed at their level of physical function (with or without *reasonable* accommodations)? Do their career goals require attendance at college? If so, do they plan to commute to a local school or live in a dorm at a school farther from home? If they are not going to college, what career path have they chosen, and how will they acquire the skills they need to succeed?

These questions are difficult for all adolescents and their families. Mobility limitations experienced by some adolescents with osteogenesis imperfecta make these questions more difficult to answer. If adolescents are unable to drive, even with adapted controls, how are they going to get to school or work? If they can drive, but require adaptations, how will the auto and its adaptations be paid for? If they require assistance with activities such as dressing or bathing, who is going to provide that assistance (especially if the adolescent wishes to go away to school)?

Strategies for building the bridge to college and/or work:
• Adolescents with osteogenesis imperfecta and their families should make contact with the state office that provides vocational rehabilitation as early as age 16 and no later than age 18, to learn about services and assistance it can provide. This agency often provides financial support for items necessary for a person with a disability to succeed in the workforce, such as wheelchair lifts for vans or specialized controls for computers and the home. It also maintains databases of important resources, such as driving instruction programs for people with disabilities and vendors who can make

modifications to homes and automobiles to make them wheelchair accessible.

• Some families may wish to also consider the assistance of a private vocational rehabilitation counselor to help with these issues and assist them with getting all the help that the state agency should provide.

• Start early in high school to contact the offices responsible for providing disability accommodations at schools and colleges to get information about accessibility of the school's campus.

• Make sure the adolescent with osteogenesis imperfecta personally visits potential schools and/or job sites to test the actual accessibility of the facilities.

As adolescents develop an adult sense of self, the desire to seek love and companionship also grows. In addition to the physical and individual moral issues relating to sexuality, as mentioned above, adolescents with osteogenesis imperfecta must be made aware of the genetic issues involved in having children. Osteogenesis imperfecta is usually transmitted to the next generation in an "autosomal dominant" fashion. This means that it is passed from parent to child in the non–sex chromosomes (autosomes), and that there is between a 50% and a 100% chance of having a child with osteogenesis imperfecta. Adolescents should receive genetic counseling so that they can make an informed decision before making a choice to have children.

Captaining the Ship

One of the biggest steps toward adult independence is leaving the home to live outside the family structure. This may occur when adolescents attend a college away from home or when they get a job that provides sufficient income to rent their own apartment. The decision to move out must be taken with consideration of the support that will be needed to accommodate the young adult's disabilities (Table 3). Issues include accessibility, support for homemaking and self-care activities, management during times of limited mobility, and getting help in emergency situations.

The farther adolescents move from home, the more they will need to rely on non–family members for support. It is probably unrealistic for adolescents with osteogenesis imperfecta to rely exclusively on roommates or

Table 3. Considerations Related to Independent Living.

Scenario	Challenges to Independence	Possible Solutions
A young man with type III osteogenesis imperfecta is independent at a wheelchair level and wants to go away to school	Getting to class Getting laundry and housekeeping done	Careful scheduling of classes to give adequate time to get to next class Hiring another student to do laundry and housecleaning
A young woman with type IV osteogenesis imperfecta who walks independently with crutches wants to live alone in a second-floor apartment	Carrying parcels and groceries up stairs	Use of delivery or Internet shopping services Ensuring that apartment building has an elevator, prior to rental, in order to transport heavy packages or wheelchair if needed for short-term use
A person with type III osteogenesis imperfecta who is dependent for lower body dressing and bathing and toileting, but independent for mobility with a power wheelchair, and who can transfer into and out of bed with a sliding board wants to live in his or her own home	Wheelchair accessibility Help for self-care activities Help in emergency situations	One-level home or apartment with doorways at least 36" wide and ramp access Personal care attendant for daytime hours Electronic emergency call pendant

college/workplace friends, since they do not have a long-term commitment to the adolescent. Thus, for some adolescents with osteogenesis imperfecta, the decision to move far from home must take into account the cost of personal care attendant services. For those adolescents, a balance of independence and support can be achieved by attending a college close to home but boarding at school or establishing an "apartment" with its own entrance within the family home.

The journey to adulthood will begin whether adolescents and their families are ready or not. It's hoped that the suggestions outlined above will make it easier to raise anchor and set sail. Adolescents need to remember that the journey is not made in one day; in fact, the journey never really ends. In keeping with the ship metaphor, it's helpful to recall that new boats go on a "shakedown" cruise before going into full operation. Similarly, adolescents should be encouraged to *gradually* take bigger steps toward independence, building on the lessons learned from previous "sails." A sure sign of success is when they are able to take the stormy times in stride as easily as the good and can cope with and learn from both.

The parents of the adolescent must allow the anchor to be raised and the ship to leave the harbor. But, just as boat builders learn from a shake-down cruise and, as needed, bring the ship in for repairs, or even dry dock, the parents should monitor the adolescent's successes and failures and be prepared to offer advice and comfort while the adolescent learns to become an adult.

May you always have the wind at your back in smooth and sunny seas, but may you also have the strength to successfully weather the inevitable storms.

CHAPTER FIVE

AQUATICS

Succeeding in a medium that supports the development of motor skills, cardiorespiratory endurance, and recreational and social competence

Holly Lea Cintas, PT, PhD

Goals for aquatics, achieving a balance in the water:
- Make a distinction between using water as a medium for therapeutic exercise versus providing opportunities for exploration, skill building, and recreational and social activities
- Describe the use of buoyancy provided by water to elicit motor skill development in anticipation of transfer to a nonaquatic setting
- Use water to provide the earliest opportunities for independent function and reinforce the infant's awareness of succeeding without help
- Map the progression from the infant's earliest kicking efforts, through stroke development and increasing independence, to becoming a skilled swimmer who enjoys being in the water

Recreational Versus Therapeutic Use of Water: When Is Each Appropriate?

Water play and swimming are fun and occur in an environment in which children with osteogenesis imperfecta can relax and excel. A recreational approach in the water encourages exploratory and playful behaviors, initiated by the child, to support a growing sense of self-competence. Buoyancy, warm water, and swim support devices initially promote comfort and relaxation, but these gradually foster a transition to increasing independence and opportunity for socialization. Depending on the child's interests and priorities (and the parents' willingness to carpool), this may lead to a range of group recreational activities, including swim team participation in some cases.

Therapeutic activities in water, supervised by caregivers, are appropriate after fractures or surgery. They can also lay the groundwork for activities that may be impossible out of the water, like kicking and walking, and can help improve cardiopulmonary function. In general, however, it is important to avoid the tendency to use the water as another exercise opportunity programmed by adults, which is often perceived as more work by the child. The infant may never gain control—and the older child loses control—of an environment that offers the best opportunity for independent movement and spontaneous recreation. To the extent possible, every effort should be made to support the infant's or child's ability to perform optimally in the water, using swim aids as needed. The objectives are to help the child to feel secure, to make independent decisions, to have fun with friends, and to pursue spontaneous recreational opportunities.

Infancy

A baby has been moving in an aquatic environment throughout the pregnancy, and warm water can provide a soothing environment for even the youngest infant. The key is to make and keep this experience positive. An uncomfortable, fretful infant will often relax when placed on the back in 1 to 2 inches of warm water in a baby bathtub with a towel on the bottom. Water has been in the infant's ears for several months preceding this, so it is acceptable if water is in the infant's ears while lying in the tub. However, if there are concerns related to water in the ears, the head can be elevated using a rolled washcloth or other soft roll. Sometimes it works well to start with the baby dressed or even wrapped snugly in a light blanket; then very gradually loosen the clothing to help the baby transition to the absence of clothing restraint. Initially this experience can be a part of the infant's bath, then can gradually transition to separate, specific activity sessions in a full-sized tub when the baby is about a month old, again with a thick, soft towel on the bottom. Water depth of between 1 and 2 inches should come to about the level of the infant's ears, which may be covered by water or not. The key is to have enough water to provide buoyancy to support the legs while keeping the face comfortably out of the water.

The first activity to encourage is *kicking* (see Chapter 2, Figure 1). Often infants with osteogenesis imperfecta cannot lift their legs or kick them when backlying on a flat surface. The legs are frequently flat, separated, and rotated outward on the support surface. Lifting the legs to kick requires the ability to bring them together, roll them inward, and lift the weight of the legs against gravity. Placing infants in backlying position in 1 to 2 inches of water (with the face out of the water) provides the buoyancy to lift the legs so the baby can kick. Usually, all that is necessary is to simply smile at or talk to infants, and they will start kicking.

The recommended frequency for doing this is twice a day for 20 minutes at a time, separate from the baby's bath. Usually it takes a few weeks to a few months to accomplish a strong kick in the water, which will gradually transition to the ability to lift the legs and kick out of the water. Once the infant can lift each leg in midline (not widely separated from the body axis or significantly rotated outward), it is no longer necessary to do the daily kicking activity in the bathtub, unless of course the baby and parents want to continue.

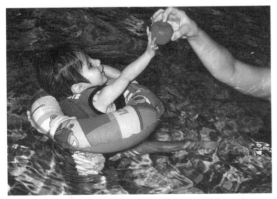

Figure 1. Reaching in the pool to strengthen the back, neck, and arms.

Promoting *reaching* in the bathtub when the baby is backlying is more challenging than kicking because reaching requires more effort from the infant. In general it is easier to begin reaching in sidelying or in a supported sitting position out of the water. However, if formatted so it's fun and not too much work, reaching can be enjoyable in the water (Figure 1). Encouraging an infant to reach from the water to grasp a toy offered by an adult may be successful once or twice if the baby is still quite weak. In contrast, suspending a toy from an overhead strap that can be batted by the infant is usually more successful. The key concept for this activity is to avoid overstimulation, read the baby's signals, and change the task as soon as it looks like it's becoming work. *Prone activities* are usually more successful in a warm swimming pool or hot tub than in the bathtub, particularly if the infant doesn't have good head control. However, this can be an opportunity to work on head control in an aquatic context by supporting the infant with one arm under the chin and chest *or* chest and armpits, and one arm under the lower trunk and upper legs. The game is to dip the baby into the water with only momentary superficial facial contact (the whole body touches the surface), and then to immediately lift the baby out again. If the baby is frightened by this, don't persist, but many infants love to do this if their threshold for it is not exceeded.

Sitting in the tub is difficult without a ring seat (see Chapter 2, Figure 8). The infant is slippery, and it's very hard work for the parent. Because of the risks associated with leaving babies sitting in the tub unattended, it has become more difficult to obtain seating devices to use exclusively in water. However, they are still available and can be useful to provide support for sitting for a few minutes in water. Keys to introducing this are timing and a careful analysis of the infant's capability in sitting. It is not necessarily easier to sit in water, so this is not the place to begin work on this activity. In fact, it is best for all concerned, especially the baby, if good head control is present, and the infant can take at least half of the responsibility for maintaining sitting on a firm surface out of the water. If this is the case, sitting in the water in a ring suction-cupped to the tub floor can be a delightful activity. Infants usually do a lot of spontaneous, interactive work with the water, thus discovering their movement capabilities and the qualities of the water through independent exploration.

Once the baby has achieved secure sitting—and this is influenced to some extent by the water level—conservative reaching activities can be introduced with a small, soft toy like a Nerf ball or rubber ducky. Reaching overhead toward a parent or to grasp an object can be a significant challenge to maintaining sitting. This is a great activity for back strengthening and alignment, but recall that an object placed too high, or too many repetitions, will extinguish this behavior quickly. Sitting in the tub offers many opportunities for creativity for parents and children. It generally works best if the child is not soapy, and sitting, as the next step, replaces kicking activities in water.

Standing in the tub can be considered in terms of advantages and disadvantages. For some children the tub is the perfect height for holding on while standing. It can be a good place to start weight-bearing in standing, using the buoyancy and weight of the water against the body to maintain the upright position. Many children without osteogenesis imperfecta do this successfully with their caregivers. Children with osteogenesis imperfecta have to be held by a caregiver positioned outside or inside the tub, depending on which position is considered the safest to support the child.

However, *the disadvantages merit very careful consideration*. At the level of the feet, it's an advantage to have them supported in early standing. This can be easily addressed by putting off-the-shelf orthotics into aquatic shoes, so the bathtub can actually become a practice area for standing when a child is too short to stand in a pool. At the level of the hips, they will typically be externally rotated (turned out), with the feet blocked against the side of the tub. In general, it's preferable not to work on standing with the legs externally rotated. However, there can be significant benefit to beginning in the water, just to give the child a feel for standing in a buoyant environment. Having the child face forward or backward in the tub rather than facing the side and holding on makes it much harder to support the child safely. Possibly, depending on the circumstances, this can be accomplished by using a harness device on the child, so the caregiver can hold the harness rather than a single arm.

Safety considerations are paramount. Once given an opportunity to stand in the tub, children may attempt this independently, thus increasing the supervisory burden for the caregiver. As the primary objective is to avoid a fall, the risks and benefits of standing in the tub must be considered in relation to the needs of each child.

Early Childhood

By the end of the first year, and often well before, young children should have sufficient head and trunk control to transition to the use of an aquatic vest or other flotation device in a spa or pool. Prior to this, holding infants or young children and swooshing them in the water is fun, but the tendency sometimes is for this to continue into the child's second, third, and even fourth year. Thus, it's an advantage for all concerned to experiment with different flotation devices to encourage physical and social independence in the water, promoting physical separation from the caregiver, who of course still supervises the child visually.

Some parents prefer to start with a small ring seat, an inner tube with a sling seat in the middle, allowing the child to ease back against the ring while supported by the seat. The advantage to this approach is that the child is physically separate from the parent, and is usually secure and comfortable if the water is warm. The disadvantage is that splashing with the arms and cycling or kicking with the legs is fun, but these don't really link to a functional stroke in the water. Similarly, placing the young child supine on a flat kickboard, held by the parent, provides the experience of being flat over the water, not held by the parent. It can be interesting, and a useful preliminary to back floating, but once

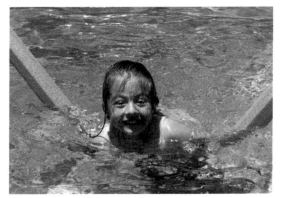

Figure 2. Use of a noodle as a support device in the water under close supervision.

again, does not lead anywhere in terms of independent effort. From these very basic flotation devices, the young child can graduate to an aquatic vest, which supports only the trunk, leaving the arms and legs free to move, or to arm inflation rings, or to a long wormlike device (a foam noodle) that goes in front of the chest and under both arms. Swimsuits also exist with flotation devices in them; some can be removed as the child becomes more comfortable in the water.

A *wide range of flotation devices* exist because there isn't a best one. The objective is to achieve a good balance between play or recreation and skill development, so it can be worthwhile to try several different devices, considering them as recreational opportunities (Figure 2). As the child becomes more comfortable and proficient in the water, time in the water can increase from only 20 to 30 minutes in the beginning to up to several hours. It's obvious that this "free time" provides not only an opportunity to be comfortable and learn to explore independently in the water, but also a peak opportunity for socialization.

In the same way a gradual transition from the bathtub to the pool or spa was accomplished, the transition from using a flotation device to swimming without one is made slowly, with great care, to ensure that the child remains comfortable, happy, and in control. Once a flotation device has been selected that allows the child to experience this medium independently, and the child is having a great time, it's time to come out of the device for brief periods to work on stroke development.

Locomotion in the water appears to be a matter of propulsion using the arms and legs. In fact, the position of the body is crucial to moving efficiently in the water. The best evidence of this is to watch a child paddle like crazy to stay above the water when the flotation device comes off. This approach often results in learning to swim, but it's the long, hard way to accomplish it. It's much easier to give the child some training in positioning the head and trunk in order to plane in the water, and then to add the legs and arms. This means teaching the child to float on the back and on the tummy.

The **back float is the best place to begin**, and young infants with osteogenesis imperfecta have already had some experience on their back in the bathtub with water in the ears. Thus, it should be a fairly easy transition from the bathtub to the pool or spa with the caregiver's hand under the child's head and bottom. If the child is nervous and insecure, one can begin in a semisitting position, caregiver's hands in the same position, then very gradually ease the child back toward full backlying. It's clear that warm water is essential to support the relaxation necessary to do this.

In the same way a diver uses the head to align the body for a back dive, a back floater learns where the head should be to keep the body close to the surface of the water. This varies considerably depending on the proportion of lean body mass to fat. Children who are lean usually have some difficulty floating. They may succeed independently only with the head fully extended backward and only the face, and possibly the chest, above the water. Children who have a fair amount of body fat can often float with the chest and trunk out of the water and the head in a fairly neutral position. Thus, trial and error experiences will be necessary to help the child become comfortable while backlying in the water, and to avoid rapid flexion of the head accompanied by sputtering and sinking.

Once the child can relax lying backward on the caregiver's hands in the water, progress can be made in two directions. One is to achieve total self-sufficiency in back floating, a significant challenge, and the other is to add kicking. It's a good idea to work on both of these directions concurrently, alternately spending some time on each. Gaining independence in back floating begins with the parent removing the hand under the pelvis, so that only the hand under the child's head remains. Often the body (not the head!) immediately goes under the water, so one should prepare the child that this will happen. This is then a good time to try some gentle kicking, emphasizing legs under the water and body extended, rather than flexing the trunk to get the feet to the surface. This is specifically not the time to work on improving the kick; that comes later. The goal is to give the child the experience of moving the body in the water as a unit, and finding the head position that permits this without sinking.

When this is progressing well, the next step is to teach the child to back float with both arms extended above the head, lying on the surface, again alternating getting used to this position with little or no external support, then doing some very gentle kicking. Floating in this position is a challenging task to accomplish, but when the child has some comfort with it, it's time to introduce holding on to a kickboard, backlying with hands above the head, then adding a gentle kick. With gentle support and encouragement that allows the child to learn these new tasks at a comfortable pace, the outcome can be the child kicking backward on the water holding the kickboard above the head with an extended body, or doing the same, arms at the sides, without the kickboard. In either case, once this is well established, it's fairly easy to work on the kick and then add the arms to improve propulsion.

Front floating with face in the water can begin during the same sessions in which one is working on back floating or other skills. It can start in the bathtub (no soap!) as well as in the pool or spa. The key is to get the face in the water in association with having fun, and many approaches exist to accomplish this. Frequently, the best way to begin is to put children in an inner tube and let them splash, so they gradually adapt to water on the face, or splash in the bathtub before using the soap. The next step might be to encourage the child to pick up water in cupped hands and splash it on the face. Wearing goggles can accelerate progress in this domain. Then, perhaps holding the nose for a quick dunk with eyes closed can be tried, then with eyes open, then without holding the nose, and so forth. Blowing bubbles in the water through the nose comes last in the progression of learning to put the face in the water.

Simultaneously with face in the water (but having fun) strategies, work on floating on the tummy begins. Unlike the back float, which is most easily learned by holding still while positioning the head to keep the face above water, the front float is learned by pushing forward in the water, often with the face out initially. This begins over very short distances, caregiver to caregiver with only 1 to 2 feet between them. The child is gently eased toward the other parent. This can quickly transition to the parent gently pushing the child toward the gutter or wall of the pool, where it's hoped the child can hold on and savor the satisfaction of having completed this independently. Once the child is enjoying these gentle pushes to the wall, the next step is to try it with a kickboard parallel to the wall, pushing the child forward, face still out of the water, giving no instructions to kick yet, but no admonition not to do so.

Once the child has accomplished the ability to plane/move forward in the water on the tummy, gradually putting the face in is added, as is the kick. It typically works best to combine two elements first, such as practicing pushing off from the parent's tummy, or possibly the wall, for short distances with the face in the water. Then, separately, pushing off toward the wall or a parent, face out, but adding a kick. All three are often then combined in the order of face in, push off, then kick. However, once again, lots of room exists for variation and experimentation. Parents and children should be enjoying this progression, that's the only strict rule.

Kicking progresses from a basic, bicycling type of pattern the infant does when lying on the bottom of the tub to a similar pattern during early attempts at locomotion on the back in the pool. In the first case, the child's body core (the back and pelvis) is fully supported by the tub, so it's relatively easy, with the buoyancy of the water, for the child to kick successfully. However, using this type of kick, the child's natural inclination while backlying in the pool, often pulls the child's body down into the water. This failure to succeed frequently makes the process of learning to swim on the back a long and tedious one. In contrast, if the child can slowly gain competence in finding the right head and body position to accomplish back floating, then gradually add the kick, this approach usually succeeds.

Two additional strategies move this process along. One is pushing off the wall backward to be caught almost immediately by the caregiver, then very gradually lengthening the distance to stay within the child's level of comfort. This links hip and knee extension with moving backward, the pattern you wish to reinforce rather than sinking at the hips. The second strategy is to practice only kicking while being supported under the back. The good news is that the same kick, a gentle wavelike arc originating from the hips, with relatively little hip and knee flexion, works for both lying on the tummy and on the back. However, this flutter kick is not natural or instinctive; it has to be learned.

Many of the same devices and positions for practicing floating can be used to practice kicking. These include hanging on to a kickboard in prone with the arms extended in front of the body, placing the chest on top of a kickboard or other flotation device, holding on to the wall or gutter, or holding on to the parent's extended arm while kicking and also perhaps putting the face into the water. What makes the swim session interesting for the child, and the caregiver, is the ability to try different things, alternating short teaching episodes with those allowing the child to do his or her own thing. Often the child will dog paddle for quite a long time after teaching has started to refine the float and stream-

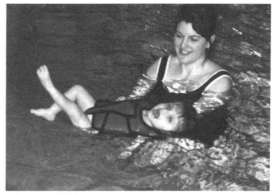

Figure 3. Kicking in backlying while wearing a support vest.

line the kick. This is not a problem, and it is particularly important to avoid correcting the child constantly. Rather, allow trial and error learning to take place so that the child reaches the conclusion that kicking with a straight body and straight legs is a much more efficient way to move through the water than the dog paddle (Figure 3).

Once the child has learned the back and front floats and has linked some form of kicking with them, one can concentrate on the ***arm strokes***, and finally, on rhythmic breathing. On the back, it's often easiest to link reaching backward with the back float and no kick, supporting the trunk from beneath until the child has some type of alternating arm stroke. Early efforts may look pretty bad, but the key is alternation rather than throwing both arms back at the same time and collapsing at the hips. Practice sessions to achieve this can occur about the same time the child is practicing kicking while going backward. When kicking is fairly well established, add the arms, and the child has the back crawl or back freestyle stroke. It may take several years, well into middle childhood, to refine this into a beautifully streamlined and efficient stroke, but if the young child can perform this in any independent form, it is a significant accomplishment.

Linking kicking, then arms, to the front float is a bit more challenging because of the position of the head and face. In fact, the child has already been working on the front float with the face out and then later with the face in the water. Pushing off from the wall, first with the face out, then with the face in, followed by kicking in prone with the face out, then face in, has prepared the groundwork for linking arms, legs, and head. Again, there are two concurrent strategies. One strategy is practicing blowing bubbles in the water through the nose, face in, followed by learning, while holding on to the wall, to blow with the face in, then rotating the head to breathe in from the side through the mouth when the face is out. Young children, depending on their interest, can learn this, but it usually requires practicing with just the face in first, then face in with head rotation to do *rhythmic breathing*. The typical mistake a child makes is to lift the head rather than rotate it, which makes the body sink, so head and neck skills require isolated practice. The other strategy to pursue at the same time is to establish front floating plus kicking, then ask the child to rotate the head to look at the elbow, then rotate back into the water with no emphasis on breathing. This cue usually helps the child learn to just turn the head, rather than lift it.

Putting these units together is again a matter of concurrent strategies. Link kicking and reaching forward with one arm at a time, with the face in, no emphasis on breathing, to help the child master kicking in extension while rotating the arms. At the same time, beginning with land drills in standing, bending forward at the waist, or while sitting, the child practices the arm stroke with rhythmic breathing. Then, only the arms and breathing are practiced while being held by a parent in the water or while standing in the water if it is shallow enough. Once the child seems to be getting this rhythm, the next step is to push off the wall or away from the parent, no kick, and practice pulling only one arm down while turning the head to that side. This then links to pushing off in a float, rotating both arms, and coordinating the breath with one arm in the water. This is frustrating and difficult, so it's a good idea to alternate it with other playful activities, and with just practicing the arm strokes and the kicking with no breathing.

Eventually, the child will get the breath in successfully, but it may take several months to put all the elements of the forward crawl together, and as with the back stroke, several years to refine it. Clearly, there are other swimming strokes to be mastered, and these will be addressed in the section below on middle childhood. However, *crawl strokes are advantageous for children with osteogenesis imperfecta for the following reasons*:

• They provide early opportunities for learning how the head influences body alignment.

• Crawl strokes incorporate repetitive hip and knee *extension* movements that are more useful for power and alignment during walking than flexion or bending movements.

• They occur with the legs together rather than spaced widely apart.

• Crawl strokes encourage back extension and elongation to promote a longer, straighter back.

Finally, the advantage of learning both front and back crawl (freestyle) strokes, and giving them equal effort, is that emphasis only on the forward crawl tends to pull the body down and forward, whereas the back crawl stretches the chest, back, and the arms backward and upward into extension. This does not mean avoiding the forward crawl altogether, rather just making certain to give equal effort to back crawl.

In addition to making progress toward learning formal strokes, independent movement can also be encouraged by encouraging young children to try a surface dive (diving from the surface of the water) to the bottom to touch it or to pick something up. Pushing with the feet off the bottom toward the surface is fun and beneficial to build strength in the leg muscles that support the body for standing on a supine stander or walking. Depending on the depth of the pool, children can sometimes walk in the water who cannot do so out of it. In these instances, walking can be encouraged as long as it does not become a burden that takes the joy from swimming and water play.

If a fair amount of walking is occurring for children who need walking devices outside the water, it might be wise to consider plantar contact (touching the bottom of the foot only) orthotics to support the midfeet during walking and pushing off the bottom. Off-the-shelf models are inexpensive, about $35, and can easily fit into aquatic shoes, which are also inexpensive. It is not recommended, unless under exceptional circumstances, that custom-made, expensive orthotic devices be worn in the pool. Among other reasons, when they are wet they cannot be put in the child's shoes to be worn home.

As described above, objectives for early childhood include becoming comfortable in the water when not held by a caregiver, learning to put the face in, floating forward and backward, and achieving some type of crawl stroke on the back and front. Rhythmic breathing, surface diving, pushing off the bottom, and walking in the water are desirable, but not crucial, accomplishments for this age group.

Gaining *endurance* in the water for young children is a matter of how long they stay in the water. It is important that the child determine this interval, which usually starts at 20 to 30 minutes and can increase to several hours. Occasionally, parents may have to insist that children get out (if they are shivering or blue), but generally the decision is based on what is enjoyable for the children, so they will want to swim again.

Pool versus spa depends on the region of the country, the age of the child, and what parents want to accomplish. For the youngest children who are not working on stroke development, it can be either, and a spa may be available in the winter so the child can be in the water year round. After a fracture or surgery, the bathtub is usually the place to begin, followed by transition to a spa or a pool, the choice of which depends on what is available and the family's preference. The temperature of the pool or spa depends on whether it is indoors or outdoors, and on the climate. The general rule is that the water should be warm enough so the child is comfortable and not shivering.

Whether socialization opportunities are better in a pool or a spa again depends on circumstances. Once the child is working on floating and kicking, a pool works best to promote more independence in the water as the child's skill level improves. Options for a pool setting vary according to location, from a neighborhood pool to adapted aquatic programs offered by some school districts, recreation centers, or Y-programs. Confirming the location by phone is the first step, followed by a parent's visit to observe whether a prospective program will be suitable before the child is enrolled. The child's interests and strengths will determine which aquatic experience is appropriate and offers the best option for lifelong opportunities in the water.

Whether or not to take *swimming lessons* varies according to the child and family. The decision to determine who should teach the child swimming is best made by the parents, who may prefer to do it themselves. However, a few private lessons can be a good investment when it is time for the child to learn specific strokes, or even to learn to be comfortable in the water while separate from the parent. Many community pools have adapted swimming programs, but they are not necessarily more appropriate than a private swimming teacher for a specific child. Conventional swimming classes are also an option when the child is highly motivated to swim and is already familiar with and comfortable in the water (Figure 4).

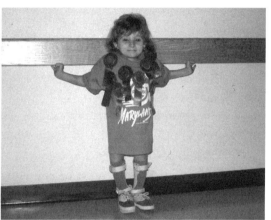

Figure 4. Swim team participation may be appropriate for some children.

Safety issues are important whenever hard surfaces are adjacent to water, so running or jumping next to the pool, spa, or soft-sided spa is risky. The possibility of unexpected enthusiasm on the part of friends or family members that could result in an injury to the child with osteogenesis imperfecta should be anticipated.

Middle Childhood

Ideally, children of school age should be independent in the pool, using a flotation device if necessary, or more typically, going solo. The exception to this would be a child who has very severe osteogenesis imperfecta, or has had a recent fracture or surgical procedure, and needs physical assistance from a caregiver to get in and out and manage in the water. For middle children or adolescents with osteogenesis imperfecta, the pool or spa is the best place to begin moving again. The warmth of the water is soothing in terms of pain, it relaxes the muscles, and the buoyancy helps the child rediscover movement for an arm, leg, or back that has been painful and immobilized. In most cases, even very young children know what to do and how to move comfortably in the water.

After a few sessions in the water with the child in charge, adult direction to work on specific movements and strengthening specific muscle groups may be indicated. Exactly what to do should be determined in discussion with the physical therapist, and clearance for certain activities may be required from the child's physician. However, it's important to move away from the therapeutic exercise perspective and toward free exploration or skill development in the water as soon as the child is pain free, for two reasons: to regain the association with the pool as a recreational and socialization opportunity, and to **work on strengthening and skill development out of the water** where the child needs to function on a daily basis. Water work is useful, comfortable, and especially valuable after a fracture or surgery, but it is not the medium in which to gain the antigravity competence essential for land function.

The child's comfort and skill level in the water are dependent on cumulative opportunities to be in the water and to practice. Children who have not yet mastered some form of forward crawl stroke and back stroke can be taught these using the linking systems and strategies described in the previous section. Those who have can refine these strokes under supervision, which brings us to considering how to do this, and the issue of safety in the water.

Families, in consultation with the child, need to make decisions about how to progress, depending on the child's and parents' preferences, region of the country, and available resources. On the one hand, there are advantages to having another adult or adolescent take over the job of coach from the parents. It fosters increased independence and gives the child an opportunity to adapt and gain comfort with people outside the immediate family, while getting one-on-one instruction. However, socialization opportunities with other children are limited with this approach. The other extreme is to sign up the child for swim lessons with age-related peers who do not have osteogenesis imperfecta. Although it offers wonderful opportunities for socialization, the risks related to unanticipated behaviors by the other children can make this approach unrealistic. So, the key is to find some combination that works for a specific child and family. One-on-one instruction will likely help the child progress more quickly, and the socialization opportunities can occur separately under close adult supervision. One teacher working with two children, one of whom does not have osteogenesis imperfecta, is another model to consider.

With guidance and supervision, the child can explore the range of available strokes, with few exceptions. Virtually any type of back stroke is acceptable and useful, the elementary back stroke being the obvious alternative to the back crawl. With the child's willing participation, practicing the flutter kick on the back (or on the abdomen) while holding a kickboard to try to accumulate distance (laps or pool lengths) is great exercise for the legs in terms of strength and alignment, as well as an excellent endurance booster.

In the same way we linked individual components above to accomplish the crawl strokes, the child can learn the breast stroke. However, there are limitations to consider. Although learning this stroke begins with the frog kick using wide open legs, pressure to transition to the whip kick is inevitable. The former is a smooth flexing of the hips and knees upward, legs widely abducted, followed by the propulsive component, extending the legs downward and together. Knees and hips are moving in the same planes. In contrast, during the whip kick, the legs are flexed upward and together, followed by a rapid rotation outward of the lower legs, generating a scooping motion of both legs. This places significant stress on the soft tissue components of the knees, which are not designed for much rotation. Given that children with osteogenesis imperfecta often have hyperflexible joints, the whip kick probably should be avoided. Learning the breast stroke is useful, and children with osteogenesis imperfecta should have the opportunity to do so, but it is not an essential skill.

Sculling, or treading water, the ability to position the body vertically in the water using the arms and legs, is essential (Figure 5). In fact, it's a lifesaving skill for anyone who is tired or fearful. Some children transition directly from the dog paddle to this, others benefit from specific instruction. The arm stroke is straightforward: elbows relatively straight, arms moving toward and away from the chest in gentle arcs. The scissors kick, a hybrid of the flutter and frog kicks, is a little more challenging. In fact, it is much easier to teach and learn the scissors kick in sidelying, as part of a side stroke, than in the vertical position. Both legs flex up, open with top leg forward, bottom leg backward, then pull forcefully together in extension for propulsion. This is an easy, comfortable kick, a nice alternative to the flutter kick, and the most efficient kick to use for sculling, a restful alternative to swimming.

Once accomplished, sculling is the easiest thing to do in the water. The butterfly stroke is the hardest. Children with osteogenesis imperfecta will see their friends doing this, and will probably want to try it. A few short strokes

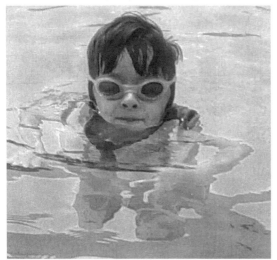

should not be a problem, but generally the *butterfly stroke is best avoided in osteogenesis imperfecta*. Advancing both arms forward simultaneously and the extreme arching of the back are very strenuous, and probably not helpful, when it is already challenging to maintain the structure and integrity of the bones of the spine. Pushing off the bottom with the feet, then doing a surface dive, pro-

Figure 5. Learning sculling and independence in the water.

vides the same porpoise type of movement, and all the joy associated with it, with far less risk.

Surface diving has been mentioned twice in this chapter, learning it initially in early childhood, and later linking it with pushing off the bottom as described above. This is safe in the absence of a collision, and it is a skill at which children with osteogenesis imperfecta can excel. Similarly, many children with osteogenesis imperfecta sit on the side of the pool, legs over the edge, to dive. Both of these methods allow the child the experience of diving under controlled circumstances. Beyond this, *diving or jumping from the pool side or a diving board are to be avoided*. It is essential to consider what the child might do when an adult is not looking, so there is risk involved in jumping or diving "just once" under parental supervision. *Walking*, if possible given the depth of the pool, can be therapeutic or used to build endurance (Figure 6). Following a fracture or surgery, the child may be able to walk in the pool long before it is possible out of water. Sometimes this can even be done using a walker in the water. The transition is obvious: when the child is able to stand and walk out of the water, the emphasis on skill development should occur there.

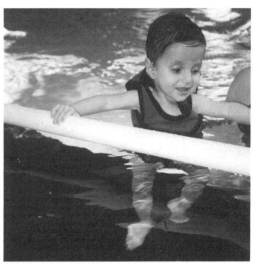

Figure 6. Walking in the water.

The exception, however, is *water walking for endurance*. The same qualities of water that provide buoyancy provide resistance to moving through the water while standing upright. Walking a few steps to several laps in the water is an excellent activity to build endurance, but it is usually more acceptable to adolescents and adults. Children frequently consider long-distance water walking an intolerable burden, and they can often accomplish the same functional gains and improved cardiorespiratory endurance while playing with their friends. Therefore, emphasis on water walking to build endurance requires consideration of the preferences of the child.

Adolescence

Achieving independence is the theme for an adolescent with osteogenesis imperfecta in all environments, including the pool or spa. For the younger adolescent, a reasonable goal is independent dressing and undressing, and depending on the severity of osteogenesis imperfecta or recent fracture or surgery, the ability to manage all activities related to getting into and out of the pool or spa. For the older adolescent, this includes getting to and from the pool independently, usually by driving a car.

As we have already noted, opportunities and objectives in the spa are quite different from those in the pool. In terms of *therapeutic exercise*, the spa is an ideal place to begin gentle movements in the presence of pain or weakness. The temperature is predictable, it may be the only warm water source in the winter months, and the socialization opportunities are obvious. The spa is useful for standing and possibly some gentle jogging (with or without an aquatic vest), but it is not the best choice for walking or swimming.

For *skill development and building endurance*, the pool is the medium of choice. It offers socialization opportunities well beyond a spa, which can be very important to some adolescents in the context of simply fooling around in the water with friends or swimming on a team. Interest in swimming varies highly among adolescents with osteogenesis imperfecta, just as it does among people in general. Children who had an early strong interest in being in the water often go on to learn several strokes that can then be refined during adolescence. This becomes the gateway for a lifelong opportunity to exercise and enjoy being in the water.

Swim team participation is reasonable for those families who wish to pursue this, but it is highly dependent on local pool access, family schedules, and the adolescent's interest in pursuing this. Most adolescents welcome the opportunity to make their own choices about what to do in the water. Often the family's most important role is to do what is necessary to help the child get into the pool on a regular basis.

There are few restrictions in the pool for the adolescent, but *diving and jumping from the side and the butterfly stroke should be avoided, as well as contact sports such as water polo*. Depending on opportunity and interest, synchronized swimming is an excellent means of building respiratory capacity and the ability to move the body in all planes in the water.

Many exercises for the legs can be done while *standing* in the water, including pushing off the bottom from a flexed position with both legs. Also, while standing, lifting each leg forward, to the side, and backward (with the knee straight) provides strengthening challenges for the muscles of the hip and knee that generalize to increased stability during standing out of the water. Kicking on the back, on the abdomen, and on the side while holding a kickboard is also valuable for strengthening and endurance purposes.

Walking in the water ranges from just starting to walk again after a fracture or surgery, possibly with a walker and an orthotic device in aquatic shoes, to endurance walking where multiple laps are counted just as in swimming. This can be a nice variation from swimming laps, but it is much more effort than most people realize, and thus an excellent cardiorespiratory challenge. *Water walking* and swimming laps are interchangeable in terms of endurance, and doing both, in addition to just having fun in the water with friends, offers valuable opportunities to enhance performance in and out of the water.

Finally, for some adolescents, the biggest hurdle to getting into the pool is achieving independence for the trip from the door of one's home to the side of the pool. It's quite easy to decide what to do once in the pool. The challenge is to focus creative thinking on the preliminaries, which can range from a van service to transport the adolescent to the pool, to enlisting a neighbor's help, to driving oneself. In some cases, overcoming this hurdle can extend to swim team participation in high school and college. These represent a few among several options, all of which can lay the groundwork for the problem-solving skills the adolescent will need following high school to function with maximal independence.

Summary: Developing independence in the water
- Kicking in the bathtub
- Sitting and swimming in the bathtub
- Wearing a support device in the pool or spa to learn to move independently
- Learning to dog paddle or swimming with any combination of legs and arms
- Learning to float on the back
- Learning to float plus kicking on the back
- Kicking on the abdomen while holding the side of the pool or with a kickboard
- Getting the face wet
- Front floating
- Front floating plus flutter kicking
- Put it together: back crawl (back float plus flutter kick, add arms)
- Front floating plus kicking, add arms (crawl)
- Rhythmic breathing at the side of the pool or with a kickboard
- Sculling as an essential lifesaving skill
- Combine front floating and rhythmic breathing (no arms yet)
- Combine front floating, rhythmic breathing, and kicking (no arms yet)

- Combine front floating, rhythmic breathing, and arms only
- Put it together: front crawl (rhythmic breathing, arm stroke, and kicking)
- Learn additional strokes as desired from a private teacher or formal classes
- Keep it fun

CHAPTER SIX

SPORTS AND RECREATION

Recreational options that promote physical activity as fun rather than work

Maureen Donohoe, PT, DPT, PCS

Goals for sports and recreation: Choose carefully, then go for it!
• Provide information on the wide range of fun physical activities that can be beneficial from a therapeutic standpoint without being formal therapy
• Identify sports and recreational activities that are relatively safe and describe what is needed for safe participation
• Describe adaptations that can enhance participation in individual and team recreational and sports activities

Physical activity is usually associated with health and fitness. When one has osteogenesis imperfecta, it can be perceived that physical activity would be unacceptable since it could make the condition worse. This is far from the truth. Physical activity improves circulation and cardiovascular fitness and allows for a sense of competition with others and oneself. It can enhance a person's abilities rather than focus on the disability. Sports are a wonderful way to be involved in enjoyable activities without even thinking about the secondary benefits gained through participation. Physical and occupational therapies are not the only safe contexts in which to work on physical activity. Formal therapy can often be complemented or replaced by more pleasurable avocational activities that provide similar physical benefits while allowing for lifetime participation in an interesting sport. With a creative mindset, people who have osteogenesis imperfecta can have fun and markedly improve their fitness through mainstream sports.

Team-related activities encourage teamwork, sportsmanship, and a sense of being part of a group. Each team member brings his or her strengths to the team to compensate for weaknesses that others may have. Team activities often require practice as a group to discover and enhance the group's strengths. Teams do not have to be made up only of people who have osteogenesis imperfecta, but can include people with a variety of diagnoses as well as those who do not have disabilities.

Not everyone has the mindset to work on a team, but many people still want to participate in physical activity. A wide variety of activities are available that allow one-on-one competition or even competition with oneself. The important thing is to become more active. Once potential athletes have had exposure to a variety of sports and recreational pursuits, they have a repertoire of activities from which to choose when looking for something enjoyable and physical to do.

Where to Start When Choosing an Activity

Once it is determined that more or different activity is the goal, the next step is to find activities in which people with osteogenesis imperfecta can participate. A wide range of activities are available, but it requires creative thinking to determine just what would be the best activity. The first thing to consider is the person's area of interest. If you do not enjoy baseball, then probably baseball would not be your activity of choice. Many families of young children with osteogenesis imperfecta report that the activities they became involved in were directly related to the child's interest and eagerness to participate in the activity.

When choosing activities, it is important to weigh the risks versus the benefits of participation. One approach can be to look for activities that address areas of deficit, such as strengthening. Another is to focus on activities that emphasize the athlete's strengths, such as eye-hand coordination. Since osteogenesis imperfecta affects different people differently, activities that are beneficial for some may be impossible for others to even attempt safely. When making choices, it is important to consider one's physical abilities and to pick sports or other activities that fit them well. The key is to become an active participant.

As with any activity, some risk is involved. When choosing a sport or recreational pursuit, consider the fracture risk before participating. Given that many organizations may be fearful of the fracture risk that osteogenesis imperfecta presents, there is a good possibility that waivers will have to be signed to absolve the organization and its players of liability if fractures should occur during participation.

Ease of participation is the hallmark of successfully beginning and sustaining a new activity. First and foremost, the activity has to be accessible. You may love adaptive skiing, but if you live in an area that does not have adaptive skiing programs, this will not be the sport you participate in on a regular basis. This is an extreme example. A more realistic example is Little League Challenger baseball. Challenger leagues are widespread and practice close to home, but teams travel long distances for games. Thus, this may be an accessible sport only if adequate transportation is available.

Physical barriers can limit accessibility to recreational options. Not all activities are wheelchair friendly. Although it may be possible to get a wheelchair on a powerboat to go boating or fishing, safety can be compromised if there are not proper tie-downs if the sea gets rough. Golf can be quite accessible for the athlete who can use a golf cart, but completely inaccessible if the course does not have adequate equipment for people with limited transfer ability to golf from the cart.

Transportation to and from activities is an issue for any person with a disability. If the athlete is young and unable to drive or manage public transportation independently, outside assistance is required to get to the activity of choice. Without a transportation commitment, consistent participation in an activity can be impossible. Some localities have solid public transportation systems that enhance accessibility to community facilities and recreational activities.

The expense of an activity can limit participation. Many activities have sign-up fees. Team sports can require expensive equipment and uniforms for the experience of playing. Usually athletes can get initial exposure to activities through adaptive sports programs, but once they're hooked, it becomes more important to have their own equipment. This allows for training at times when the group is not available to practice. Most important, having one's own equipment allows for the equipment to be adapted specifically to individual needs.

For athletes who have a higher than average risk for injury due to osteogenesis imperfecta, another important consideration is to have a support system when participating in recreational or sports activities. Someone should be available to provide first aid if necessary. It is helpful for people who have transfer challenges to designate someone who is aware of the special needs of people with osteogenesis imperfecta to be available to assist with transfers. This could help to avoid fractures even before the activity begins. Sometimes it is necessary to have a one-on-one aide to modulate the activity, enhance the experience, and retrieve items that cannot easily be recovered without help. This support person can be a parent or a volunteer who has been trained in the special needs of that athlete. For the very young child who is participating in a recreational activity, the support person tends to be a parent or a classroom aide.

Once the potential athlete decides physical activity is a goal, and an area of preference is established, it is time to find available resources. The first place to investigate is local resources. Local recreation centers, schools, Little League, Special Olympics, rehabilitation centers, and boat clubs are wonderful places to start. Often, the local community offers activities that can be easily adapted for those with osteogenesis imperfecta.

The Internet is another great place to investigate resources for activities. Searching for adaptive sports or for specific activities opens a world of opportunities. The National Center on Physical Activity and Disability at http://www.ncpad.org has a great Web site with categories including health promotion, sports programs, and equipment suppliers. There are many links to help the athlete learn more about specific sports of interest. The National Sports Center for the Disabled at http://www.nscd.org has a site that details winter and summer activities. These sources of information and others listed in Chapter 8 can be helpful in developing an idea of what recreational activities might be interesting to the potential athlete.

Guidelines for Participation

When choosing an activity, the athlete must consider risks versus benefits to determine safe participation. The activity should be easily adaptable to the special needs of someone with osteogenesis imperfecta and should promote the goals of the participant so that, first and foremost, it is enjoyable. The sport should draw on some of the athlete's strengths. Activities requiring concentration and eye-hand coordination often appeal to people who have good cognitive skills. If the goal is strengthening, look for activities that place an emphasis on strength. If cardiovascular fitness is the goal, choose activities that encourage participation for longer durations. If the goal is to just get outside and do something, there are plenty of activities that could be suitable for those with osteogenesis imperfecta.

Much of this chapter is devoted to examining the benefits of specific activities, then addressing the drawbacks or risks of participating in them. It is imperative that people who have brittle bones avoid full contact sports. This means that even if you have an undying passion for rugby or tackle football, the risks outweigh the benefits, and full participation should be avoided. This doesn't mean you can't manage the team or keep score or record the statistics, but active participation, including refereeing, should be avoided. Moderate-risk activities appropriate for a younger child when support staff is present to modulate the activity can become inappropriate when competition becomes fierce in the teen years and beyond. A good example is basketball, which is not very aggressive when young children play but can be quite dangerous when adults play pick-up games or when groups of children with varied diagnoses play wheelchair basketball. This does not mean that a teenager shouldn't go outside and shoot some hoops, but it does mean that formal competition in the teen years may be contraindicated.

Activities involving unpredictable rotational stresses should be avoided. Gymnastics is an example of a noncontact activity that could be potentially dangerous for the athlete with osteogenesis imperfecta. Although it involves some very positive benefits of building strength and flexibility, several aspects are very risky, including the need to get into positions that are not functional. Specifically contraindicated activities include somersaults, cartwheels, and back bends. Balance beams, vaults, and uneven parallel bars are some of the equipment used in gymnastics that can also put a person at risk of fracture.

High-impact activities should be chosen carefully. Marching, long-distance running, long-distance hiking over uneven terrain, high-impact aerobics, activities involving jumping, and many forms of martial arts can place a person at unnecessary fracture risk. Even people who do not have brittle bones can develop stress fractures when participating in these activities.

When looking for an activity, consider the things addressed above, including expense, accessibility, potential enjoyment, and support personnel. Be creative in the approach to physical activity. Encourage others to help make it possible and it can happen.

Physical Education in School

The role of physical education in school is to give children exposure to other children in a recreational context and to activities they can participate in throughout a lifetime. Physical education should help children establish good exercise habits so that they maintain a healthy level of activity not only during gym class but through adulthood. That said, many youngsters with osteogenesis imperfecta are often left on the sidelines during gym class. The reasons include the school's (and possibly the parents') fear that the child could be injured during class activities, the teacher's limited ability to adapt activities to be appropriate for a child with osteogenesis imperfecta, and the class's limited ability to modulate the level of activity to be safe around a person who fractures easily.

Since physical education is mandated in 47 states, it is important that children and adolescents with disabilities have the opportunity to participate in appropriate physical activity as part of the school curriculum. This does not mean being the scorekeeper for every contact sport encountered in gym class, nor does it mean having physical therapy in lieu of gym. It means that young people with osteogenesis imperfecta should take part in a physical activity that is geared to their strengths. The gym class also should enhance the repertory of physical activities available to the child in the process of learning lifelong fitness.

Adapted physical education is for students who, for whatever reason, are unable to participate safely or successfully in regular physical education. Placement in adapted physical education is a judgment call and is determined according to where students can most likely achieve their physical education potential. Since physical education is supposed to teach lifetime skills, an established adapted physical education program also teaches children how to adapt activities to allow participation in the future. Everyone involved with children who have osteogenesis imperfecta should have knowledge of safety limitations during physical activity. They are responsible for helping children learn their safe boundaries in a given activity.

Adapted physical education practices vary widely. Unfortunately, practice and service can range from exemplary to terrible. In some cases, a teacher specially licensed in adapted physical education teaches students who can benefit most from such an approach outside the regular physical education setting; in other cases, someone with no specific, formal adapted physical education expertise might teach similar students.

Quite a few activities can be an appropriate part of a typical gym class. These include fitness activities such as basic calisthenics (sit-ups, toe touches, flexibility exercises). Depending on the child's level of ability, push-ups and modified pull-ups can be acceptable. Participation in a walking or wheelchair propulsion program is a reasonable fitness-related activity, depending on the child's level of skill and interest.

Floor hockey is an easy activity to adapt for children with osteogenesis imperfecta. The sticks tend to be made of foam and are light in weight and easy to manage. For a child using a wheelchair, the stick can easily be taped to the wheelchair to allow active participation in the sport. When playing from a wheelchair, it is sometimes helpful to start out with a larger ball so the child can develop the skill necessary to maneuver the chair and hit the ball simultaneously. Once the skill is developed, the size of the ball can be progressively reduced.

Many physical education classes for young children include scooter board activities. As long as the child is closely monitored so the scooters do not become bumper cars, these activities have many benefits for those with less severe osteogenesis imperfecta. Scooters can be propelled from a sitting position as well as when the rider is lying down on belly or back. Scooters can be a great strengthening activity and can even promote cardiovascular fitness when performed for extended periods without stopping. Before this is organized as a group activity, the child should have experience with the scooter board and it should be determined that the child has the strength and balance to maneuver the scooter board safely.

Although not every school has a pool, when one is available, swimming is an excellent fitness-related activity that can be performed during gym. If the school has access to a swimming pool, parents should encourage the school to emphasize this activity in the child's physical education.

Tether ball is a playground activity that can easily be adapted to allow safe participation. This game is typically played with two participants. A firm ball similar in size and weight to a volleyball is attached to a rope that is attached to a pole. The ball is batted back and forth between the two opponents with the use of hands or forearms. The game is won when the rope is completely wound around the pole or when the opponent fouls out of the game. Fouls are caused by hitting the ball with any body part other than hands and forearms, hitting the rope, catching the ball, throwing the ball, or winding the rope too low on the pole (typically lower than the 5-foot mark). This game is easy to play from a sitting or standing position and it can be adapted by using a lighter ball, such as a beach ball. Wrist and elbow guards similar to those used for roller skating could be used for added safety by the player with brittle bones.

Creativity is the key to success with adapted physical education. The American Alliance for Health, Physical Education, Recreation, and Dance at http://www.aahperd.org is a good resource for parents who need help in defining physical education and adaptive physical education goals when advocating for their children. It is an up-to-date resource on health-related legislation in the United States. The Web site http://www.pecentral.org offers ideas and techniques for adapting physical education for teachers, parents, and students.

Lifetime Recreation and Sports Activities

The activities discussed below have a five-point star (*) system assigned to each entry. Developed by the author of this chapter, the star system is set up with risks and benefits taken into account. One star shows low risk/benefit, five stars indicate high risk/benefit for a specific activity. Risks include physical contact, rotational force, high velocity activity involving the athlete's movement or an object coming toward the athlete, repeated movements that could cause stress fractures, and fall risk. Benefits include strengthening, improving flexibility, improving cardiovascular fitness, enhancing eye-hand coordination, and allowing for a sense of sportsmanship as an individual or team member.

Aerobics

Risk factor: ★★★   Benefit factor: ★★★★

Aerobic exercise classes became very popular in the 1980s and continue to appeal to many people. Typically these classes are set to music and involve dance routines designed to increase a person's heart rate. The wide array of aerobic classes includes high-impact aerobics, low-impact aerobics, step classes, cardio kickboxing, spinning, and aqua aerobics. Pilates exercises also could be included. Many classes can be adapted to accommodate the various needs of those who have osteogenesis imperfecta. The key is to find an appropriate class and work with the instructor to help meet individual needs. If aerobic classes are not easily accessible, an exercise video can be adapted to allow activity that is beneficial for cardiovascular endurance. This is a noncompetitive, noncontact activity that promotes exercising with a group.

There are many benefits of participation in an aerobic exercise class. These classes are designed to help improve cardiovascular fitness. Most classes also have a flexibility component that will address the hamstrings, hip flexors, hip adductors, Achilles tendon, and sometimes the lower back. These self-stretches, if performed correctly, can be an excellent adjunct to a daily exercise routine, even when not in class. Many classes have a strengthening component with emphasis on the arms as well as leg strengthening for antigravity activity, including the gluteal, quadriceps, and abdominal muscles. This strengthening can be helpful for improving posture in sitting and standing along with enhancing function in these positions.

There are some areas of risk with aerobic activity. High-impact aerobics and activities involving rapid changes in direction and difficult moves can increase fracture risk. The experience level of the teacher can be a negative influence on the safety of the exercise. Some instructors have very limited education prior to teaching an exercise class. It is very difficult to know in advance if the instructor has a wide range of exercise experience, including knowledge of the needs involved with a specific diagnosis of osteogenesis imperfecta. The instructor may have no experience and may have developed an unsafe program for those who do not have physical limitations, let alone someone who has brittle bones. Thus, it is important that the class participant be aware of the potential risks related to exercise classes. It is essential to listen to your body, make your own decisions, and not always do exactly what the instructor is doing. Remember that the goal is activity and movement, not pain.

People with physical limitations due to osteogenesis imperfecta may need to adapt the exercise class to their specific needs and limitations. For an ambulatory person who fatigues easily, it can be helpful to bring a chair to class so that sitting while exercising is an option as fatigue increases. If moving on and off the floor is an issue, and the class performs these activities, it can be helpful to discuss with the instructor how frequently floor exercise is necessary in class. If it occurs once, at the end of the class, and there is assistance to perform the transfer, it may be feasible to perform the activity with the class. If there is no help for the transfer or floor activities are interspersed throughout the class, the instructor can be helpful with exercise alternatives for the participant.

If the participant uses a wheelchair for most activities, it may be unreasonable to expect to do floor activities. The easiest adaptation is to perform the arm movements or to propel the wheelchair in the same directions as the class is moving. It may be helpful to look into classes that are geared toward older people when looking for an exercise class. These classes tend to be paced a bit slower and include moves that require lower impact. Some geriatric classes are specifically designed for exercise while sitting and therefore need little or no adaptation for wheelchair users.

Archery

Risk factor: ★★★   Benefit factor: ★★

Archery is a sport that involves using a bow and arrow to shoot at a target or other object. It is an Olympic and Paralympic sport as well as a hunting activity that depends on eye-hand coordination and upper extremity strength. For athletes with osteogenesis imperfecta, this sport is most safely performed at the entry level, with a relatively light bow and the string at low tension. The risk of injury increases with the use of bows that are larger, heavier, and have higher tension. Athletes must consider their baseline strength when deciding if archery is an appropriate sport. Entry-level target competition bows require 25 pounds of strength to pull the string. This is not easily accomplished by many people who have osteogenesis imperfecta, but it would be feasible to use a lighter noncompetition bow. The arm that stabilizes the bow is at greatest risk of injury when participating in archery. That arm supports the bow while the other hand pulls the string to release the arrow. As the string recoils, it can snap back on the forearm and cause bruising and even fractures in more significantly affected participants.

This sport can be adapted by mounting the bow on a surface support so that the shooter aims and draws the string but does not have to deal with the weight or recoil of the bow. This is more commonly done for archers who use a crossbow for hunting. There are many Web sites dedicated to adaptive bow hunting for those who have limited arm use. The site set up by the Buckmasters American Deer Foundation has an extensive array of possible adaptations to make crossbow use universally accessible. It can be reached at www.badf.org/ disabled_hunters/adaptiveequip.html.

Baseball

Risk factor:★   Benefit factor: ★★★★

The Little League's fastest growing division is the Challenger division. This program enables every child to participate in a structured athletic program, regardless of ability level. In Challenger games, "buddies" are assigned to help their challenged partners around the base paths if assistance is necessary. Many times, these buddies are typically developing children who enjoy baseball. The Challenger division is the Little League's way of providing new opportunities for children with disabilities so that everyone can get into the game.

This team sport has minimal physical contact with the other athletes. It is an activity where the emphasis is on ability rather than disability, and the coaches strive to adapt things so that all who play can be successful.

As in any ball sport, there is always the risk of getting hit by the ball, which could cause a fracture. For those who walk and run, there is risk involved in running for the bases and fielding, but this risk is no higher than that involved in everyday activities on the playground. Unfortunately, Challenger baseball has not expanded to form adult leagues, so there is a limit to how old one can be to participate, and this activity is not available in every community. If the team is local, there may be a travel requirement to allow competition with other teams. Many teams are large and diverse enough that if there are not adequate numbers for a Challenger league, there are enough members to split the team to allow competition.

To find a Challenger baseball team, contact the local Little League or check out programs on the Little League Web site at www.littleleague.org.

Basketball

Risk factor: ★★★   Benefit factor: ★★★

Basketball involves getting a ball into a hoop that is suspended above a court

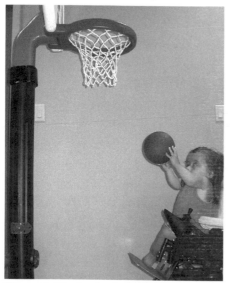

or other surface. The nice thing about basketball is that it can easily be played at home or in the community. It is an activity that can be started from a very early age with a toy basketball set and a reduced-size ball (Figure 1). As a child grows and gains skill, a net that can be raised to regulation height can be used outside of the home with a regulation-size ball. This is an activity that is regularly found on the playground, and basketball leagues for early elementary school children are not uncommon.

Figure 1. Playing basketball.

This activity involves eye-hand coordination to get the ball into the basket as well as upper body coordination to dribble the ball across the court. A certain level of strength is required to pass the ball. Basketball is an enjoyable activity that can be played with family and peers from an early age and emphasizes overhead reaching and trunk extension. It can be played from a sitting or standing position.

Although this is a very accessible and accepted sport, basketball becomes less safe for those with brittle bones as they get older and with more players in the environment. In the early years of competition, the players are well protected by the coaches and referees since all the players are learning the rules. As children get older, the competition becomes tougher and there are increasing risks of injury during the game. The same is true with wheelchair basketball. Opponents and teammates in wheelchair basketball can tend to be a bit too aggressive for a person who has brittle bones to play on a team safely. This does not mean that once competition becomes too tough, it is no longer a sport in which to participate. It means that the activity changes with age. It is relatively safe to shoot hoops with peers and family members who understand osteogenesis imperfecta and therefore can modulate the activity to a safe level.

Billiards

Risk factor: ★   Benefit factor: ★★

Billiards is a table sport that involves using a stick (a pool stick) to hit a ball (the cue ball) that will hit other balls and, it's hoped, direct those balls into a pocket and off the table. The most common activity in billiards is pool, or pocket billiards. Bumper billiards, with pinball-like bumpers on special tables, is also available. The most common game of pool in the United States is eightball, in which there are actually nine balls to be shot off the table. The balls are numbered one to nine. The goal of the game is to shoot all of the balls into the pockets until just the eightball remains. Billiards can be played individually, but it is most commonly played competitively with another person or in team pairs.

Billiards does not require a great amount of physical strength or endurance but does require good eye-hand coordination. If one does not own a pool table, it is relatively inexpensive to rent one in a public venue. This is an activity that can be performed from a sitting or a standing position. The pool stick is light in weight and does not require the participant to get into positions that would increase the fracture risk.

This is a low-risk activity since it does not rely on a great deal of physical strength or endurance. Placement of the table can limit access to those who rely on a wheelchair for mobility. For the pool shark who is ambulatory but is short, as well as for wheelchair users, some tables can be too high to easily make all available shots. The creative ambulatory pool player can try standing on a chair or stepladder, but this increases the risk of injury when playing and is therefore not advised.

Boating

Risk factor: ★★   Benefit factor: ★★★

Boating can allow for active participation, including managing the boat, steering and propelling the boat, or just enjoying the ride. A wide range of opportunities are available to a person who has osteogenesis imperfecta, including adaptive rowing programs, canoeing, crew, kayaking, powerboating, and sailing. The level of active participation is often directly related to the size of the boat. The smaller the boat, the more likely the passenger is also responsible for managing the boat.

Adaptive rowing programs are designed to allow people with disabilities to learn boating skills with the goal of competition (Figure 2). Initially, the disabled rower is coupled with an ablebodied rower in a two-person oar boat. Boats can be adapted with outriggers to increase the stability of the boat, therefore reducing the risk of tipping. Since the boater sits inside the boat, there are specially designed seats to provide support through the lumbar spine if necessary.

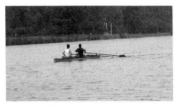

Figure 2. Adaptive rowing involving a mixed pair.

If the rower is able to use leg strength, seats can have a sliding component that allows for a total body workout of arms and legs with each stroke. The one drawback of the sliding seat option is that the feet have to be strapped into the seating device. This can cause increased risk of fracture if the lower limbs are asymmetrical in alignment or length.

Adaptive rowing allows for competition between rowers of similar ability. Regattas have classifications for boats containing mixed pairs where one rower is able-bodied as well as classifications for single rowers who have varying levels of disability. Competition and practice are held on rivers or large lakes that do not have a strong tidal influence or currents. World Rowing has more information on adaptive rowing that can be accessed at http://www.worldrowing.com.

Canoes are narrow boats that carry one to three people. One paddler in the front of the boat and one in the back, who is also responsible for steering the canoe, typically propel these boats. Given their narrow width, canoes are relatively easy to tip over when someone is getting into or out of them and when they are used in strong currents. Some canoes are designed for passengers to sit on the bottom and others that are slightly wider are designed to have the paddlers sit on seats attached to the boat's crossbars. It is more stable to sit on the bottom of the boat but easier to transfer into and out of the boats with seats on the crossbars.

Canoeing allows for travel in waters that are relatively shallow. Although canoes can also be used in waters that have rapids, it is not advisable that a person with a high fracture risk participate in canoeing in fast water or rapids. This is a sport that can be done purely for recreation, but again, it can be competitive. If one does not own a canoe or live near an appropriate body of water, canoes can often be rented at lakes and rivers on which it is safe to travel. Organized canoe trips can be found that range from paddling for several hours to paddling over several days, which can include camping out at night. Canoeing uses upper body strength and promotes cardiovascular fitness. It is an activity that relies on repetitive motions that are self-limiting.

Crew is a competitive boating activity that allows for one, two, four, or eight rowers to propel a boat, or shell. The rowers sit in the bottom of the boat on a seat known as a slide and have their feet strapped into the foot stretcher. Depending on the type of shell, the rower can use one or two oars. One-oar rowing, also known as sweep rowing, occurs with two, four, or eight rowers. Two-oar rowing, known as sculling, occurs with one, two, or four rowers. Rowers are expected to row as a unit so that each rower is doing the same aspect of the stroke at the same time. This can be difficult for an athlete who has asymmetrical strength or alignment or both. Boats that have four or eight crew members can have a coxswain who is responsible for calling the strokes for the rowers. These team members ride on the shell facing the rowers and keep the pace of the rowers in line. The best coxswains are small in size so that the weight of the boat is minimally increased, but they must have strong verbal skills. An athlete of small stature who has osteogenesis imperfecta can be an excellent adjunct to an able-bodied crew, especially since monitoring the boat's progress and direction during racing and practice has low risk for injury.

Kayaks are small, narrow boats created for one or two people to paddle. Paddlers sit in the boat in a long sit position. Sea kayaks are designed with a hole in the top that the kayaker sits in. A skirt can be added to seal the opening around the kayaker so that if the boat is capsized it does not fill with water and can be uprighted with minimal difficulty. An ocean, or sit-on-top, kayak is open, which allows for the boat to self-bail easily when hit by a wave. Inflatable kayaks, which are more like ocean kayaks than like sea kayaks, are another option. All kayaking is managed with a double-edged paddle that is held in the center and dipped into the water on either side of the boat to propel it. Kayaking can be done on a wide variety of waterways from gentle streams to white water to oceans. It is safest for those with brittle bones to choose calm waterways on which there is minimal risk of tipping the boat.

Powerboats vary in size from very small ones that accommodate two people to very large cruise ships with multiple decks. The boating experience needs to be in line with the type of experience desired and available to the boater. Although some small powerboats are able to go into rough seas, this may not be a safe activity for those who have limited mobility. The same boat in calm waters can be perfectly safe.

Smaller powerboats require that passengers sit inside the boat. Therefore, wheelchair users must transfer out of the chair to get into them. Given the size of the smaller boats, they are usually easy to steer and learning how to manage them is relatively easy.

As boats get bigger, the need for assistance in managing the boat increases. It is not uncommon to be just a passenger on a larger boat. These boats can be used for transportation, such as a ferry, for recreation, such as a fishing boat, or for relaxation, such as a cruise ship. Larger boats that have multiple decks may have limited accessibility since doors are frequently not flush with the floor but have a step of a few inches to manage. Not every boat with multiple decks has an elevator. Historically, stairs on small ships are tall and narrow and therefore may be difficult to manage. Exposed stairs such as those out on deck can have the added problem of being slick from the sea air and weather. Care must be used when moving throughout the boat.

Like powerboats, sailboats vary from small boats that one or two people sitting inside can manage to large schooners that can sleep many people. Smaller sailboats require a person in a wheelchair to transfer into the boat. The sportsman in the stern (the rear of the boat) is responsible for steering and managing the sail. This activity is quite accessible for a boater with good upper body strength. Catamarans with two pontoons and a flat trampoline suspended between them are sailboats designed for ocean use. These sailboats may not be very safe for a person with brittle bones since it is sometimes necessary to hold onto the boat in rough seas and possibly lash oneself to the boat.

Larger boats vary with respect to accessibility. Sailboats that are large enough to walk around on may also be able to accommodate a wheelchair. It is important to note that when planning on sailing while in a wheelchair, the boat must have some form of tie-downs to prevent the chair from moving unexpectedly. Larger boats are often ridden for pleasure and skippered by someone with diverse sailing experience. It is quite doable for a person with osteogenesis imperfecta to learn how to steer and navigate a larger sailboat, but the risk of fracture increases significantly if managing the sails and moving across slippery decks becomes an aspect of sailing. For more information on adaptive sailing, check into US Sailing at http://www.ussailing.org.

Boating has many benefits, but they vary with the type of boat that is chosen. All aspects of boating allow the sportsman to experience nature and enjoy the water. Boating can be used for recreation, sport, or transportation. It can be competitive, with racing possible in many kinds of boats. A boat can be used for vacation cruising or simply be the place where other activities like fishing are performed. Boating can bring independence to those who are capable of managing a boat such as a kayak or small powerboat without support personnel. The use of oars and paddles in boating allows for upper body and trunk strengthening as well as cardiovascular fitness while participating in an enjoyable activity.

Given that boats bobbing on water have moving surfaces, there is always some risk when transferring to a small boat, whether the person is ambulatory or in a wheelchair. Once aboard, there is risk of tipping in rough seas on a small boat or risk when moving around on a larger boat in the same conditions. Caution must be used when moving around on boats because of slick surfaces and possible water on the decks. Smaller boats, canoes, and kayaks often have to be removed from the water and stowed or transported when the activity is finished. Assistance may be needed for this since handling these boats out of water can increase fracture risk.

Larger boats that allow boaters to walk or wheel onto them may be easier to access but there may be unanticipated obstacles. Boats that have stairs for access may be inaccessible to wheelchair users while others that have ramps may not have ramps wide enough to accommodate a chair. Access is a consideration that should be investigated prior to the planned day of boating. If the boat is on tidal waters, the access ramp will change in angle in response to the tide. Ramps can be very steep and not negotiable without assistance at certain times and relatively flat at others.

All boaters should wear life jackets. Those who are at increased risk of fracture should be careful choosing an appropriate floatation device. The vest should completely surround the boater rather than have a single strap that crosses the back. The vest should be secure and snug, but should not impinge on the ribs if tugged upward. The same action should not allow the device to be pulled up past the boater's ears.

Those using small boats such as kayaks and canoes, which have a risk for tipping over, should wear a helmet and possibly even elbow pads. This will protect against major injuries that could occur during unexpected impacts.

For those who have difficulty getting onto or near the ground and need to transfer into a small boat, a two-step transfer box can be helpful to allow scooting down. This box can be created to be a few inches shorter than wheelchair height at the top step with the bottom step a few inches from the dock. The boater scoots down the steps and then into the boat, requesting assistance as necessary.

Boats that allow wheelchair access should have tie-downs for safety. Tie-downs similar to those in vans can be installed on the deck of a boat with minimal difficulty. On calm seas it may not be necessary to use the tie-downs but if the seas are rough or if the sportsman is also fishing from the boat, tie-downs help improve safety.

A good place to search for more information on wheelchair-accessible boating is to investigate adaptive fishing. Some companies have specially adapted pontoon boats that are easily accessible and require no transfer skills.

Cheerleading

Risk factor: ★★★★   Benefit factor: ★★★★

Cheerleading allows spectators to become active participants in the venue of contact sports that they cannot play directly. Cheerleading has become a sport in itself, given the gymnastic and dance skills incorporated into the basic cheers that were once heard on the sidelines. This activity requires strong vocal skills, an advantage for many people with osteogenesis imperfecta. Although someone with osteogenesis imperfecta may not be in the middle of the intricate choreography and throws that are sometimes seen, cheerleading can be easily done from a wheelchair when the emphasis is on verbal rather than physical skills (Figure 3). At most schools there are try-outs for cheerleading where the cheerleaders are judged on their cheers, jumps, presentation, voice, and spirit. It is a competition of skill and ability.

If cheerleading is a passion for a person who has osteogenesis imperfecta, it is important to discuss with the coach the assets you would bring to the team prior to the tryouts. In this way, judging does not have to emphasize jumps but can emphasize spirit, knowledge of cheers, voice, and knowledge of the sport. One nice thing about cheerleading is that accessibili-

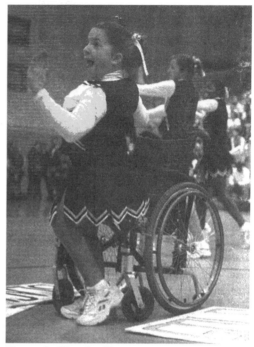

Figure 3: Cheerleading.

ty is usually not an issue since being on the sidelines for basketball, football, and soccer games rarely entails managing stairs.

Drawbacks related to cheerleading involve safety on the sidelines of a contact sport. Cheerleaders have to be ever cautious of stray balls, and other athletes, that may come at them unexpectedly. For cheerleaders who are on their feet performing the same repetitive movements as their teammates, it is important to understand there is a risk of stress fracture in the long-duration repetitive movements common in cheerleading dance routines. The gymnastic activities cheerleaders are known for represent a great risk for those who have osteogenesis imperfecta. Despite their small stature and ease of being lifted, persons with osteogenesis imperfecta are strongly warned against participating in activities that involve being lifted, carried, or thrown for the sake of the team's choreography. Gymnastic routines are not acceptable activities in the realm of cheerleading for those who have a higher than average fracture risk.

Cheerleading squads that are open to having a member with special needs have accepted the responsibility of adaptations prior to the athlete's participation. Adaptations can include minimal changes, such as not having the athlete directly participate in the gymnastic routines but having the cheerleader artistically involved in the routine. Some cheerleaders can do well with shock-absorbing insoles in shoes for when repetitive dance steps are expected. Athletes who use alternative mobility devices may need special assistance for accessibility as well as a more creative choreographer for cheerleading routines.

Cycling

Risk factor: ★★   Benefit factor: ★★★★★

A wide range of cycling experiences are available to the general population. These can be divided into two categories, stationary cycling and overground cycling. Stationary cycling is most commonly done indoors with a cycle that stays in one place. It can be an upright cycle or a recumbent cycle that is lower to the ground and has a seat that includes a back support. Some stationary cycles include components that allow arm exercise simultaneously or instead of lower extremity use. Most stationary cycles have adjustable tension to allow pedaling with little or no resistance or a great deal of resistance, depending on the rider's strengths and needs.

There are even devices that can convert a typical cycle into a stationary cycle. This may seem like a cost-effective option but it is important to consider the stability of the cycle once it is converted as well as the amount of resistance the cycle provides. Usually resistance is not adjustable and sometimes the stationary adaptation provides so much resistance that it is nearly impossible to pedal.

In some rehabilitation catalogues there are inexpensive sets of pedals available that can be set up in front of a chair to allow pedaling with use of arms or legs. These relatively inexpensive exercise cycles usually have few or no adjustments for tension and therefore frequently give no resistance when pedaling. This type of cycle can be an option for someone who has limited transfer ability but has a desire to exercise with equipment.

Cycles designed to be used over the ground come in a variety of shapes, sizes, and price ranges. When choosing a cycle, it is important to consider present strengths as well as future goals for the equipment's use.

Entry-level bicycles are small and often have training wheels for added stability. These bikes usually are fixed-gear models and have coaster brakes. On the next level, bicycles have gears to allow three, five, ten, or more speeds to ease the ride over rolling terrain. These bikes have hand brakes. Training wheels can be added to these bikes if necessary, but they typically are not designed for the extra set of wheels. Bicycles with gears can be categorized as road bikes, mountain bikes, or hybrids. Road bikes are lighter, narrow, and have smooth tires that work well on paved surfaces. Mountain bikes are shorter than road bikes and are broader in the frame as well as the tires. The knobby tires of a mountain bike are designed to ride more comfortably on unpaved surfaces. This type of riding is not safe for a person who has a high fracture risk since the chance of falls increases with off-road riding.

Hybrid bikes are wider than a road bike but narrower than a mountain bike. These bicycles are designed to travel mostly on paved roads but occasionally over unpaved surfaces for short distances. The handle bars are designed to allow the rider to sit more upright than the bars on a road bike. This type of bike is a good option for someone who is looking for a stable bike that can be ridden on the road but whose emphasis is not on speed.

Bicycles designed to be ridden in a reclined position are called recumbent bicycles. These two-wheeled cycles are low to the ground, have a bucket seat, and the pedals are in front of the rider. Recumbent bicycles have several drawbacks. Currently only adult-sized models are available, and these may not be acceptable options for those with short stature. The bikes are rather unstable and can be easily tipped over, so if a recumbent bike is an interest, it might be advantageous to try a recumbent tricycle, which is more stable, lessening the risk of falls.

Tricycles are often thought of as cycles for the very young. Inexpensive tricycles can be found in most toy stores. Careful assessment is necessary to make sure the purchase is low to the ground with a wide base for limited tipping risk during turns. Unfortunately, many tricycles are poorly designed, tip over very easily during turning, and should be avoided for young children with osteogenesis imperfecta. Young children may be more secure on a model with big wheels or a low to the ground cycle with a seat that has a back. Stable tricycles (or three-wheeled bicycles) of various kinds are available for people of all ages who require more stability when riding.

The typical tricycle has the pedals attached to the front wheel so that when the rider stops pedaling, the tricycle should also stop moving. This is called a fixed-gear cycle, in which there are no options for variation of resistance on inclines or level surfaces. As the tricycles get larger and more expensive, they will also have chain-driven wheels so that the pedals are not directly attached to the front wheel and the force is generated through the rear wheels. These tricycles are easier to pedal over rolling terrain than the front wheel direct-drive tricycles. Chain-driven tricycles can have either coaster brakes or one hand brake for the rear wheels. These tricycles have the ability to coast on downward inclines, unlike the front wheel direct-drive tricycles. Chain-driven tricycles can be found in upright and recumbent models.

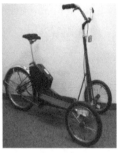

Figure 4. A Step 'n Go cycle.

Some adaptive tricycles allow the rider to use both arm and leg strength to propel them. Although this appears to be a great way to get a total body workout, the arm and leg components are directly related, so that the arms and legs must be working at the same speed at all times. This is not necessarily safe for a person who has unequal strength because of fractures and immobilization of one or more extremities. These tricycles are not recommended for people who have osteogenesis imperfecta unless the arm and leg components can function independently.

The Step 'n Go cycle is a relative newcomer to the tricycle scene (Figure 4). It is a tricycle that allows the rider to stand or perch on a seat with feet on treadles. As the rider shifts weight from one side to the other, the cycle is propelled forward. This type of cycle allows a person with unequal leg length or limited range of motion to ride a cycle and therefore gain the benefits of cycling that were not available previously because of physical limitations. The cycle is useful in rehabilitation since it incorporates weight-shifting and lower extremity strengthening. The rider can work on the normal weight shifts necessary for walking after fractures while maintaining a modified weight-bearing status. These cycles can be ordered with a variety of options, including fixed gears or multiple gears, a Whoa Bar that a support person can utilize while walking alongside a rider to control unsafe movement, antitipping wheels for the back of the cycle, and even adapted brakes for those who have limited strength for braking. For more information on this cycle, the company's Web site is http://www.stepngo.com.

Handcycles are another type of cycle available to those who have limited power in their legs but who have good upper body strength. A wide variety of handcycles are available, with just as wide a price range. For children, there are two types of hand-driven tricycles. One is a typical tricycle that has had the crank adapted so that instead of using foot pedals, there is a chain attached to the front wheel that attaches to the hand crank. The other type of pediatric handcycle has a seat that is separate from the frame of the trike so that the child does not have to straddle the tricycle. This too has a hand crank that is chain-driven from the front wheel. As the cyclist outgrows pediatric cycles, several options become available. Basically, the choice depends on the cyclist's size and ability to transfer. Most models are close to the ground and require the athlete to straddle the handcycle. Some cycles allow for the legs to be flexed while others support the limbs in an extended position. Adult and large pediatric models of handcycles are available with a bench seat that does not require the rider to straddle the cycle. These cycles have a higher center of gravity and therefore are not necessarily designed for competition. It is very helpful to try all types of handcycles before investing in a piece of equipment. A resource on the Internet for those who are interested in handcycling is http://www.handcycle racing.com.

Many benefits come from cycling. It is a wonderful form of transportation. It works on cardiovascular fitness as well as muscle strengthening. Cycling can be helpful for improving range of motion of the extremities that are used in pedaling. Cycling allows for peer-related activities for people with less severe osteogenesis imperfecta Cycling opportunities for competition are available in adaptive sports programs. A growing arena for handcycle competition can be found in able-bodied races that are half or full marathons and that also include wheelchair racers. For those who are younger, tricycling using stable devices is often available to preschoolers and children in early elementary school gym classes.

The key to getting involved with cycling is to use equipment that meets the needs of the rider. If the rider is new to the sport, the most stable equipment is important, such as a nontipping tricycle, a big-wheel model or other low rider, or a bicycle with training wheels. Riders should be able to easily touch their feet to the ground when a bicycle comes to a complete stop. This is not imperative when using handcycles or a Step 'n Go because these are designed to be stable with a rider in place when the cycle is stopped. Equipment with a poor fit or that is not appropriate for the rider's skill level will put the cyclist at unnecessary risk of fractures.

The risk of impact with another cyclist or a car is always a factor. The choice of riding venue can affect the safety of the riding experience. High-traffic areas create greater riding risks than closed biking trails that have no motor vehicle access. Off-road mountain biking presents a significantly higher risk of falls than does road biking. This is not a great choice for a person with brittle bones and should be avoided if possible.

To improve safety when riding, it is important to use a well-fitting helmet and pads. Gloves with a gel palm pad and elbow pads may be helpful to protect the extremities from unexpected spills, although it is critical that wrist guards or leg padding not restrict the mobility necessary to ride safely. An extra set of wheels can help increase stability on a bicycle or Step 'n Go. If the cyclist has questionable balance and skill on the bikes, these extra wheels, often known as training wheels, can be helpful in limiting the risk of falls. If a tricycle or low rider is being used by a person with limited unsupported sitting endurance, seat adapters can be purchased to give the cycle seat a back. These can be found in adaptive equipment catalogues.

For those who intend to use a cycle as a means of transportation and who rely on assistive devices such as crutches or a walker for ambulation, it is important to consider how to adapt the cycle to manage the assistive device. It is great to get from point A to point B but if you are lacking support to walk on arrival, cycling becomes an ineffective mode of transportation. A simple adaptation can be to attach a piece of large-diameter PVC (polyvinyl chloride) pipe to the back or side of the cycle to hold a set of upright crutches. No adapters to attach crutches or walkers to a cycle are commercially available, so creativity is important when coming up with a solution. If the cyclist has difficulty transferring down to the level of a handcycle or a recumbent bike, a two-step transfer box can be fabricated to aid in the transfer. This box would allow the cyclist to transfer out of a wheelchair, sit down to a comfortable level, and then scoot down one step to be level with the cycle. The reverse action is performed to transfer off of the cycle.

Dancing

Risk factor: ★★   Benefit factor: ★★★★

Dance can be as structured or as free as the participant's interest. Many adults in this world consider themselves excellent dancers but have never had a dance lesson. The key to dancing is to enjoy the music and move your body with it. Dance can be as formal as ballroom dancing and ballet or as free form as modern dance and the latest movements performed on music videos and in dance clubs.

Some dances are not safe for those who have brittle bones. Modern dancing, which requires some aspects of gymnastics and can be a high-impact activity, is not advised. Tap dancing, which requires repetition while in shoes that have very poor shock absorption, can put a dancer at risk for fractures. Break dancing is contraindicated because of the high rotational forces involved and the fact that it can sometimes be considered a contact sport. Dances that require frequent turns and rotational forces, such as the tango or ballet, should be approached with caution. Jumping activities should always be approached with caution and avoided if possible.

The age of the participant is helpful in determining the appropriateness of dance classes. Ballet is a fine activity if performed with caution for the young ambulatory child, but as the emphasis on form increases, it becomes a less appropriate activity. Those who have osteogenesis imperfecta must remember that there is an increased bias for the hips to be rolled outward, or externally rotated, in ballet. Although ballet encourages this posture, it is not advantageous for those who are at risk for bony deformity. When participating in ballet at an early age, the emphasis should be on learning dance steps and the basics of ballet, which include strength, balance, and flexibility. These aspects should be performed within a comfortable range but should never be forced. As the challenges of ballet move into dancing on point and leaping, it becomes a less acceptable dance form for the child who has osteogenesis imperfecta.

Ballroom dancing, performed with a partner, can be a low-impact activity. For ballroom dancing, the dancer with osteogenesis imperfecta must choose a partner who is keenly aware of the physical limitations and who will work as a team to protect against fractures while dancing. This includes not stepping on toes when learning a new dance step as well as not running into other dancers on the dance floor.

A growing area of performance dance is adaptive dance, the pairing of a nondisabled dancer and a wheelchair user. This has brought to the public the fact that people who use wheelchairs can be as graceful, creative, and artistic as the nondisabled population. The adaptive dancing Web site at http://www.adaptivedancing.com has more information on wheelchair dancing with an able-bodied partner.

Dancing has many benefits. It is a very inexpensive mainstream activity that can be performed just about anywhere there is a source of music. It works on cardiovascular fitness if the dancer is participating for several minutes at a time without stopping. It can work on strength and flexibility while encouraging positive peer interaction. The dancers do not have to be able to stand or walk to participate; all they have to do is feel the rhythm and move their bodies in ways that feel good.

The risks involved with dancing relate directly to the type of dancing and the environment in which it is performed. A crowded dance floor has more risk of impact injuries than an empty living room. Dances that require twists, turns, and frequent repetition place the participant at greater risk than those that do not require them.

Dancing requires participants to be creative and open-minded about the activity. This is an activity that does not have to be put on hold when a bone is casted; it just changes to adapt for the cast. Adaptations for dance are an extension of the creative endeavor, so just feel the music and move!

Fishing

Risk factor: ★★   Benefit factor: ★★

Fishing can be as easy as dropping a line with a hook in the creek down the street or a full-scale, deep-sea fishing trip in search of big fish. The fishing experience that an outdoorsman seeks is related to desire and accessibility. Fresh-water fishing usually uses lighter weight equipment than its cousin, ocean fishing. Fish caught in fresh water also tend to be smaller and therefore easier to manage than the fish caught while deep-sea fishing (Figure 5). Fly fishing is often done on moving streams or rivers and can be done from the shore or while wading in the water. Fly fishing while wading is the one aspect of fishing that is not encouraged for people with osteogenesis imperfecta. The risk of falling is substantial when walking on slippery rocks in running water.

Fishing has many benefits. A successful fisher is able to supply a food source. It is a sport that can be relatively inexpensive but can grow to be as extravagant as the sportsman's interest in the activity. Fishing can be a relaxing day outside with friends or it can be an active day at sea, reeling catches in. Those who are creative and have good finger dexterity may enjoy tying fly-fishing lures on days they are not out fishing. Casting is a great activity for promoting upper body strength and range of

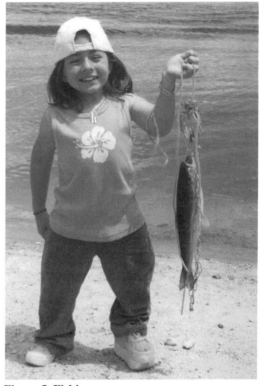

Figure 5. Fishing.

motion. Reeling fish in is not only great for enhancing a sense of accomplishment but is also a wonderful strengthening activity.

Unfortunately, fish are unpredictable, and fishing can be risky. Until the fish is hooked and out of the water, it is not known how big it is and how much it will fight being caught. It is helpful to have an assistant when a fish gives a significant amount of resistance. This assistant may complete the reeling-in process or may just stand by to net the fish once it is out of the water. When fish are caught, they often bring water out of the sea with them. This water is left surrounding the fisher and can be quite slick. It is important to be aware that surfaces that were once easy to negotiate can be unsafe when wet from a day of fishing.

Adaptations for fishing include pole holders that anchor the rod on the ground or boat when fishing for extended periods or reeling a fish in. As noted above, it is helpful to have a fishing partner to help manage reeling in and netting aggressive fish. This partner should be considered a fishing friend rather than assistant since it is always more fun to fish with a friend on days when conversation is more plentiful than fish. More information on adaptations for fishing can be found at Fishing Has No Boundaries, Inc: www.fhnbinc.org.

Golf

Risk factor: ★★   Benefit factor: ★★★

Golf has recently exploded as a sport of interest for all ages. This is a sport that basically involves hitting a small ball with a club with the goal of getting it into a cup set in the ground. Golf is a sport typically performed outside on a full-sized golf course, which has 18 holes, or at a miniature golf course, which tends to have 9 holes. Two skills are needed for golf: driving and putting. Driving is a forceful hit of the ball to make it travel far distances, and putting is a softer tap of the ball to get it traveling short distances and into the cup. Putting is easily accessible from a standing or sitting position. It is the basic skill needed for miniature golf. Driving requires rotatory forces of the body in order to control the direction and distance the ball travels. The feet are often planted firmly and the rotation comes from the trunk and shoulders. Driving ranges are public places where people can practice their golf skills. At this type of facility no walking is required since it is basically a place to hit balls at targets.

Golf requires a moderate level of swinging, bending, balancing, and sometimes walking that in turn helps to build strength, flexibility, and stamina. Golfers do not usually share these aspects of the sport as much as they expound on how great it is to be outside on the course and how wonderful it is to get the ball in the hole. Each golf course is designed to be a beautiful outdoor environment. Often the beauty created includes the challenge of the game when getting balls past sand traps and water obstacles.

Although golf has many benefits, risks are involved in an activity that requires rotational forces. Driving is not an activity appropriate for everyone with osteogenesis imperfecta. Some golfers who have less severe osteogenesis imperfecta may have no problems with this forceful action while others should not attempt it. Those who walk the course should be aware that the terrain can be uneven, and therefore they must use caution. Not all courses are accessible for those with special needs. Assistance will be needed for managing the weight of a golf bag full of clubs. This may entail getting help to put the bag on the golf cart or even hiring a caddy to manage the bag for the golfer. Those who have transfer issues may have difficulty with participation, but many of these issues can be overcome by a motivated golfer.

The United States Golf Association has a resource center for people with disabilities that can be accessed at http://www.resourcecenter.usga.org. A variety of adaptive carts are available so the golfer with standing and transfer difficulty does not have to move out of the cart to be successful with golfing (Figure 6). A caddy can be a helpful adjunct to the golfing experience, even if a golf cart is used. The caddy can be responsible for selecting the various clubs for the golfer, minimizing the risk of fracture associated with managing a golf bag.

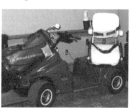

Figure 6. An adapted golf cart.

Hockey

Risk factor: ★★★   Benefit factor: ★★★

When one thinks of hockey, the vision of a person with osteogenesis imperfecta does not usually fit in the uniform. Hockey is associated with rough play that occurs often while the participant is on ice skates or roller blades. Players use long wooden sticks to push a hockey puck on ice or a ball on land across a field into a goal. Similar activity occurs with field hockey where the stick is not quite as long and the interaction is not quite as rough. Still, ice hockey, street hockey, and field hockey tend to be too aggressive for a person with brittle bones.

For those who enjoy the sport, there are options. Floor hockey is a sport that has been adapted for gym classes. It involves a lighter plastic or foam stick that is used to propel a plastic puck across a floor. This activity can be adapted to allow sticks to be attached to wheelchairs. Since this is a slower and less aggressive activity than regular hockey, it is relatively safe.

A relative newcomer to the sports scene is sled hockey, or sledge hockey. It is played mainly by people with various lower extremity disabilities (those with amputations, spinal cord injuries, cerebral palsy, or post–polio syndrome, for instance). The player uses arm strength to propel a sled by digging the picks on the ends of two short hockey sticks into the ice, pulling the sled forward. A right stick and a left stick (the blades are curved differently) are used that are miniature copies of a typical hockey stick, except for the metal picks (like figure skate toe picks) on the ends. With the sticks, players shoot, pass, and propel themselves.

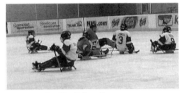

Figure 7: Sled hockey.

The players sit on the sleds, which are affixed to two elongated hockey skate blades under the seat. The sleds are about 3 inches off the ice and are anywhere from 2 to 4 feet long, depending on the size of the player. The sled glides on the blades and a metal bar in the front. For beginners the blades can be set wide apart for stability. The player, who wears the same padding a typical ice hockey player would wear, is strapped into the sled with multiple straps to maximize control of the sled.

The few differences between a sled hockey game and a typical hockey game are these: 15-minute instead of 20-minute periods, two sticks instead of one, and the sled hockey players sit on a sled rather than stand. The puck and the pads are regulation hockey equipment.

The benefits of participating in hockey include that it requires teamwork, encourages strength and agility, and works on cardiovascular fitness. There are aspects of eye-hand coordination involved in shooting the puck to a team-mate or into the net.

As expected, hockey, especially sled hockey, is a high-risk sport. Players all wear chest pads, elbow pads, and helmets with face guards. Participants who are at high risk for injury wear a special colored helmet (such as bright orange) so the other players know this is not a player who can have physical contact. A penalty is given to the player and team if the high-risk athlete is checked.

For more information on sled hockey, visit the US Sled Hockey Association Web site at www.sledhockey.org or Sledge Hockey of Canada at www.shoc.ca.

Martial Arts

Risk factor: ★★★   Benefit factor: ★★★★★

The martial arts encompass a range of movements and self-defense styles. As an individual sport that allows athletes to progress at their own pace, the focus is on what you can do, not what you cannot do. Since many of the martial arts are geared toward self-defense, they emphasize kicks, punches, and throws that would not be safe for a person who has brittle bones. These include judo, jujitsu, wrestling, akido, and hapkido, which all require participants to be thrown by their opponents. On the other side of the spectrum is tai chi, a Chinese martial art that focuses on controlled movement. It involves a series of fluid movements known as forms.

Most martial arts fall between the high-risk throwing activities and the low-risk forms of tai chi. Karate, tae kwon-do, kung fu, and kempo are additional examples of martial arts that use punching, blocking, and kicking to defend and attack. However, like tai chi, they emphasize structured forms that combine attacks and blocks to produce a choreographed defense against multiple attackers. Balance, strength, endurance, speed, and flexibility are required to correctly perform the forms. Each form progresses in difficulty but students have the freedom to move at their own pace.

Adaptive karate classes are available in some communities for those who have physical disabilities. These classes do not focus on the contact aspects of martial arts but work instead on balance, breathing, coordination, flexibility, strength, and self-control. These classes usually have a low teacher-to-student ratio and frequently have a physical therapist or an occupational therapist helping out with the class to address specific performance needs of the students. Although it may be difficult to find an adaptive karate class, if there is a strong interest by the student, some studios will develop a special program for a very motivated student. It is important to remember that if a person has brittle bones, kicks and punches can be done into the air rather than into a bag when working on skill.

Research on the benefits of tai chi for older people documents that compliance with a program results in reduced falls. It is felt that each movement allows one to divide attention to the performance of the form while also focusing on balance and weight shift. This can in turn help to improve awareness of one's surroundings when not exercising. There is also a marked improvement in fitness, strength, and blood pressure with the use of tai chi. Although there are no studies related to osteogenesis imperfecta and tai chi, these benefits can be advantageous for a person who has increased fracture risk.

As with any sport that requires time spent on one foot, there is a risk of falling while participating in martial arts. The athlete must remember that this is not a competition with other participants but an activity that enhances individual balance skills and strength. The emphasis should be on working within a safe range; therefore, kicks or punches into the air should never meet an object or person. Those who use a wheelchair will have the benefit of experiencing the holistic aspects of the sport but should not become frustrated with their own physical limitations.

Making phone calls and networking is quite helpful in finding an appropriate martial arts class that meets the needs of a person with brittle bones. Some classes are geared to people with special needs and therefore the training routines can be performed as a group. Other classes have instructors who require one-on-one training to ensure safety and appropriate adaptation, while other instructors are just not able to address the specific needs of individuals with physical challenges. It is helpful to screen facilities, possibly watching a class in action or participating, to avoid signing up for an inappropriate class. Avoid facilities that require patrons to buy into lengthy (and sometimes expensive) contracts until it is established that this is an activity the athlete will enjoy pursuing for an extended period.

Racket Sports
Risk factor: ★★★   Benefit factor: ★★★★
Racket sports can be helpful to build upper extremity strength and agility. Although there are many benefits, not all racket sports are created equal. Sports such as lacrosse, racket ball, and squash have a high incidence of contact-related injuries and are therefore not good choices. In contrast, table tennis, badminton, and tennis have beneficial qualities that outweigh the negatives.

Table tennis is also known as Ping-Pong. It utilizes a light-weight paddle and a light-weight ball that is hit over a net attached to the center of a table. This is a sport that can be played in singles or pairs. It is also possible to practice independently. Ping-Pong is an Olympic and Paralympic sport. In the Paralympic Games there are a variety of levels at which the athlete can compete, given the level of function. Table tennis can be played from a sitting or standing position and is therefore acceptable for a wheelchair user as well as a person who is ambulatory. However, playing while standing can require quick body shifts that increase the risk of fracture.

Tennis and badminton use a larger racket to hit a ball or a birdie over a net to an opponent. As with Ping-Pong, both sports allow for singles or doubles to play against opponents. The tennis racket is heavier than the badminton racket. Both are mainstream sports that can be played with minimal set-up in a public court or in a back yard. The court surface may have an impact on participation. Tennis can be played on clay or grass courts, while badminton is most often played on grassy surfaces. A clay surface is much more predictable for an athlete moving on foot or in a chair, although a grass surface can be more forgiving if falls occur. Tennis requires a ball that has a tendency to roll away if it is not hit and that could hurt a player if it makes contact with the athlete rather than the racket. Badminton uses a birdie that is light in weight and does not roll away. A birdie does not generate the same speed as a ball and therefore has a lower risk of causing injury to the athlete. Wheelchair tennis (Figure 8) is a growing sport that can be found at many rehabilitation centers large enough to have community programs. For more information, www.wheelchairtennis.com is sponsored by the International Tennis Federation and provides rules, regulations, and tournament notices.

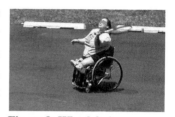

Figure 8: Wheelchair tennis.

Racket sports are a wonderful form of one-on-one competition. They can be as aggressive as the athlete is capable of being. Equipment is inexpensive and there is minimal set-up necessary. Participation in racket sports helps improve upper body strength while working on eye-hand coordination. For those participating from a wheelchair, racket sports can help improve wheelchair agility skills. If the athlete is able to stand and walk, racket sports are helpful in improving walking and possibly running speed. All racket sport players have the opportunity to enhance their reaching skills during play.

Racket sports tend to be fast paced, so there is a risk of falls when moving and changing directions rapidly. Uneven surfaces such as grass courts can increase the risk of falls and possible fractures. If a ball hits the athlete, it could cause bruising and even fractures in more fragile athletes. The bending required to retrieve balls and birdies can be stressful for some athletes. If this is a problem, reaching devices can be helpful to increase accessibility and prevent unnecessary stress on the joints.

To get started with a racket sport, adaptations are sometimes helpful. Table tennis can be played on a surface smaller than a regulation-sized table so that the athlete can learn how to serve and return the ball without getting frustrated.

Tennis can be set up as a tether ball activity. For those who are just starting out managing a racket and a ball, it is helpful not to have to run after the ball on a regular basis. If the ball is tied to a pole or a fence, it can be hit and then easily retrieved. Starting with a larger ball or balloon and working down to a regulation-sized ball is also helpful when learning this skill. Once the athlete has a good understanding of how to hit the ball, it can be gently volleyed between opponents as greater skill is developed.

Skiing

Risk factor: ★★★★★   Benefit factor: ★

Skiing has the benefit of allowing the athlete who enjoys being out in nature in cold weather to participate in a widely accepted sport. There are some well-established, cost-effective adaptive skiing programs throughout the country with support staff well trained in adapting ski experiences for people who have a wide variety of limitations. These programs allow people with physical limitations to meet and socialize with other like-minded persons, although the chances of finding another person with osteogenesis imperfecta on the slopes may be rather small. Adaptive skiing works on balance, agility, and strengthening. Minimal cardiovascular benefits can accrue for the novice skier, but as the participant becomes more independent in skiing, the fitness component increases.

There are many risks and drawbacks to adaptive skiing. First and foremost, it is an activity in which it is difficult to control speed. Additionally, controlling the level of experience of the ski program trainers who are assisting the skier as well as the able-bodied skiers on the mountain is an extreme difficulty. This is a high-risk sport for fractures and not an activity one could take up without extensive training and planning.

Although many adaptive skiing programs function at minimal cost to the skier, there are transportation, lodging, clothing, and lift ticket expenses. This is not a sport that can be achieved without a strong support system to help with transfers (onto and off the ski lift and into and out of the ski apparatus are just two areas) and equipment management. Additional help is needed for tethering the skier, clearing the slope to ensure skier safety, and supplying first aid if necessary from any area of the ski resort. If the athlete becomes invested in skiing, the equipment needed for adaptive skiing can be very expensive, especially when purchasing one's own. Transporting this equipment becomes another dimension to consider.

In order to be successful in adaptive skiing, the safest piece of equipment is the mono-ski with outriggers, which allows the skier to sit and use weight-shifting through the trunk to help move the ski down the hill but minimizes the risk of falling. When using this device, the skier needs to wear a full helmet that includes padding at the neck, as well as body padding similar to that worn by those who would participate in ice hockey. In general, because of the high fracture risk, adaptive skiing may not be appropriate for many individuals with osteogenesis imperfecta.

For more information on adaptive skiing equipment, check Disabled Sports USA at www.dsusafw.org.

Swimming

Risk factor: ★   Benefit factor: ★★★★★

From the time a child is diagnosed with osteogenesis imperfecta, swimming can be emphasized as a fitness activity for a lifetime. Please refer to Chapter 5 for more information on swimming and other aquatic pursuits.

Wheelchair Track and Field

Risk factor: ★★★★   Benefit factor: ★★★★

Track and field events may be referred to as wheelchair athletics. These can be divided into wheelchair racing (both short- and long-distance events) and throwing events. Throwing events include the shot put, javelin and discus throws. In shot put the contestants attempt to throw (or put) a ball (or shot) as far as possible. The ball is the heaviest of the objects thrown, weighing more than 5 pounds. It is typically balanced on a shoulder and thrown with one hand. The discus is a flat object, weighing less than 2 pounds, that is thrown toward a target. The javelin is a long pole, weighing 1 to 2 pounds, that is thrown for distance. All throwing activities require a great deal of upper body

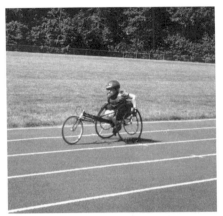

Figure 9. Wheelchair track racing.

strength and rotational force to gain throwing advantage.

Wheelchair racing is a growing sport (Figure 9). It can be done from a standard wheelchair but as the athlete gets more involved with the sport, it is helpful to have specialized equipment to maximize speed and endurance. Many specialized wheelchairs are available specific to the type of racing the athlete prefers. Short-distance racers on tracks tend to use a wheelchair that is not as long or as low as the wheelchairs used for long-distance races over city streets (like marathons).

Wheelchair athletics emphasize strength, endurance, and coordination. These activities are individual sports but they can be dedicated to a team. This means that athletes who are aligned with a team generate points for the team as they win individual events. Practicing for wheelchair racing involves little set-up, if the athlete has a chair that has a low center of gravity. People involved in wheelchair sports tend to have average or above average cognitive status and are very dedicated to their sport.

As with any sport, there are risks involved. Throwing sports require a high level of rotational force to generate the power of the throw. Although the item being thrown may be relatively light, the physical adaptations necessary to propel the item can put a person at risk of fracture. Many athletes stabilize their bodies on special field chairs or in their own wheelchairs in order to enhance the throw. Although this amount of stabilization improves the outcome, it also increases the torque across the thrower's legs and trunk, increasing the risk of fracture. Firm stabilization of the body to enhance the power of a throw is not advised for athletes who have osteogenesis imperfecta. Therefore, throwing sports may not be a wise choice for most athletes with this condition.

Wheelchair racing has risks because of the potential for impact with another chair, cyclist, car, or pedestrian. One must consider that the faster the wheelchair is moving, the more unstable the chair becomes when it moves over uneven terrain or around corners. This risk of tipping is important to consider, even when using specialized chairs that are designed for speed. Helmets, arm pads, and wrist supports can minimize the risk of injury, but cannot prevent it. Overuse injuries of the upper extremities are possible for endurance athletes. It is helpful to consult a coach who is well versed in proper technique to learn good habits when embarking on this sport. Good training early can help prevent long-term injuries that could limit participation.

Parental Influences

Children with brittle bones often have parents who have become quite apprehensive over time about activities that could put their child at risk for fractures. There needs to be a balance in the family that allows the parents to be supportive of the child's activities but not put the child at risk of fracture. Most parents of children who are active in sports and recreation report that their child was the driving force behind the child's participation. When the child does participate, the parents ultimately become the advocates. This involves informing the activity group as to what things are safe for the child.

As in any sports activity, parents will have to sign waivers that relieve the organization of liability if their child should get hurt. On rare occasions, parents must fight for their child's participation in physical activities because of the fears of liability of the particular organization. Once involvement is accepted, the parents become the first aid team and the transportation. This is a huge commitment. Parents often report that it is all worth it, however, to see their child happily participating with other children in activities the child loves.

Sometimes children are not self-motivated to participate in sports or recreational activities. Often this is because they have not discovered activities that bring them enjoyment. Parents of these children have a harder job since they often have to overcome their own fears of their child being harmed before they feel comfortable about encouraging safe recreational activity.

When Accidents Occur

When athletes are involved in physical activity, it is not uncommon to have injuries. It is of the utmost importance that an athlete with osteogenesis imperfecta is well prepared prior to participation for any unexpected accidents. Precautions taken to help prevent injuries include judicious choices of appropriate recreational activities, and possibly the use of helmets and padding. Although this equipment does not always protect against fractures, it is helpful in minimizing injury. The next step for minimizing injury is to have a support person designated to take the lead if an injury occurs. The support person should have a general knowledge of how to splint an extremity. He or she should also have a bag packed with emergency splint materials, a cell phone or access to a telephone, parental permission for treatment if the athlete is underage and the parents are not present, and the athlete's insurance cards.

If a fracture is suspected in an extremity, it is important to listen to the child with osteogenesis imperfecta, not to move the extremity too much, and not to attempt to reduce the fracture. The extremity should be immobilized with firm stiff material on either side of the bone including the joint above and below the suspected break. This splint should be gently secured with Ace wraps or other wrapping material. Some medical facilities supply families with emergency splints made out of thermoplastic material that can be used to immobilize an extremity in case of emergency.

Once the fracture is immobilized, it is important to call the child's orthopedist to get recommendations on the next step for medical management. If a trip to the emergency room will result in an x-ray of a known fractured bone but the athlete will have to wait until the next day for the bone to be set, it may be advantageous to just make the appointment with the child's orthopedist and wait for the next day if the splint is managing the limb effectively. However, a limb that has been rodded and has a risk of the rod protruding or being broken has to be x-rayed at the earliest possibility because surgical intervention may be needed. Additional information about fracture care is available in *Growing Up with OI: A Guide for Families and Caregivers*, Chapter 2: First Aid, available from the Osteogenesis Imperfecta Foundation, Gaithersburg, Maryland.

Injuries that involve loss of consciousness or suspected cervical (neck) fractures are a medical emergency requiring immediate attention. It is important to notify the emergency system so that the athlete is transported on a back board with the head and neck immobilized in an ambulance. When a cervical injury occurs, it is important not to move the athlete except as necessary to ensure the person is able to breathe until emergency medical personnel arrive.

In general, the joy of sports and recreation far outweighs the risk of injury for the majority of children with osteogenesis imperfecta. Careful choice of appropriate activities, proportional to the child's level of ability and interest, is obviously important, as is the need to teach other children in the environment about the condition so they can learn to respect the special needs of children with osteogenesis imperfecta.

Special thanks to Karen Turner-Bare and Betsy Mullan for editorial assistance, and to Bob Wellmon and Jason Beaman for sport-specific assistance.

CHAPTER 7

DEVICES AND EQUIPMENT

Their role in facilitating performance while enhancing safety and engaging children

Joanne Ruck-Gibis, PT, MSc, and Kathleen Malone Montpetit, OT, MSc

Goals for adaptive devices and equipment:
- Outline the general categories of equipment that can be useful at various stages of development
- Describe equipment and devices that promote safety, early mobility, independence, and optimal body alignment, reduce the caregiving burden for parents, and meet the aesthetic and social needs of families
- Describe how the adaptive equipment and devices recommended can improve the quality of life for children with osteogenesis imperfecta, their parents, and siblings

The devices and equipment mentioned and pictured are for illustration only; inclusion does not imply endorsement.

The use of appropriate adaptive equipment and devices can improve the performance and ultimately the independence of the child with osteogenesis imperfecta. Exploration and experimentation at all stages of development are essential ingredients for independence. The challenge is to encourage meaningful activity while minimizing the risk of fracture and increasing the child's sense of accomplishment. These are the key elements if the child is to achieve independence in gross motor skills, self-care, and mobility.

Devices and Equipment for Use in Supine (Backlying)

In the early stages, infants with osteogenesis imperfecta are comfortable in the supine position and are often placed in it. Our goal with this position is to facilitate head turning, reaching, kicking, and rolling to the side. Unless fractures make it necessary to place infants or children on the back, however, sidelying is chosen over supine.

When infants or children are obliged to spend time on their back, using towel rolls to promote symmetry of the

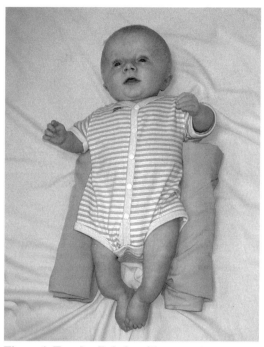

Figure 1. Towel rolls help with symmetry.

legs, arms, and head is suggested (Figure 1). This technique avoids an exaggerated rolled out and flexed position of the hips. As soon as the infant demonstrates some ability to move either the arms or the legs, the support should be removed to stimulate active movement of the limbs.

Toys to encourage reaching and kicking in supine

To promote reaching in supine, suspend mobiles consisting of colorful sponge balls or soft squeaky toys overhead close to the baby's arms. Reaching for them can help strengthen the baby's shoulders and elbows as well as develop eye-hand coordination. Interest in the toys facilitates a symmetrical head posture and strengthens the neck muscles as the baby turns to look and reach.

For older infants, the same method of placing a mobile overhead is beneficial for stimulating leg movements, which activate hip, knee, and ankle movements. Colorful booties with bells encourage kicking and hand-to-foot movements, which in turn strengthen muscles of the neck, abdomen, hips, and shoulders.

Devices and Equipment for Use in Sidelying

To encourage sidelying, a rolled towel or receiving blanket placed behind the back can be used to bring the young infant very gradually toward sidelying, beginning with only 15 degrees at first and gradually increasing the angle until the sidelying position is obtained. For some infants simple, inexpensive commercial sleep positioners, such as head-hugger sleep supports, made of foam wedges or rolls can be custom cut to hold the young baby in sidelying. These are available at most comprehensive toy stores. However, it is crucial to ensure that a foam device does not come in contact with the infant's face or obscure the infant's breathing.

When in sidelying, it may be necessary to start with a rolled washcloth between the knees, then gradually decrease the thickness of the washcloth until none is required. Some families use an elastic stocking to hold the legs partially together for this purpose; however, this interferes with the baby's ability to move independently and may not be advantageous for hip development. The stocking should not be used for long periods but can be used in therapy. It is usually possible to bring the legs together fairly quickly if the baby's position is changed frequently from backlying to sidelying.

Sidelying is the easiest position in which to start work on reaching because the arms move in a gravity-neutral plane. To promote reaching and to keep the infant's interest, place musical or visual swipe toys close to the baby so that interacting with them requires little physical effort initially, reinforcing success in reaching in sidelying.

The most effective toys for these goals are the cause-and-effect type that light up or make a noise after being touched. Another suggestion is toys that are light and easily batted, and that squeak when touched (toys for cats, for instance). Even an infant with significant weakness is able to elicit an effect with these toys.

Many parents ask about using soft baby carriers (Figure 2), and some are useful to encourage sidelying. If parents wish to use a carrier, one that promotes sidelying across the parent's chest using an asymmetrical shoulder strap is recommended. This position is preferable to those in which the baby is straddled symmetrically over the parent's chest with the legs widely abducted (open) and flexed. Forward- or rear-facing soft baby carriers or hard backpack carriers are not recommended until the baby demonstrates good head and trunk control enabling postural adjustments while in the carrier. Prolonged sitting in these carriers (for more than 30 minutes without a change in position) with hips open and rolled out (abducted, or externally rotated) can promote sustained, undesirable alignment for the legs and back. Furthermore, be aware that backpack carriers take the child out of view of the caregiver.

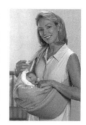

Figure 2. A soft baby carrier.

Devices and Equipment for Use in Prone

Infants with osteogenesis imperfecta frequently do not have sufficient head control to lift the head and free the face in order to breathe when placed prone on the tummy. Devices used to promote movement in pronelying are not appropriate until infants achieve such head control (see Chapter 2 for strategies designed to develop this skill). Commercially available mats with visual, auditory, and tactile stimuli can encourage movement and exploration in this position (Figure 3). One example is the 1-2-3 Discovery Lane Playmat.

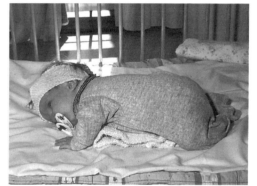

Figure 3. A stimulating crib environment.

The earliest locomotor efforts on the tummy often consist of the infant moving backwards, sideways, or in a circle. In the same way that appropriate choice and placement of toys can elicit reaching in sidelying, infants can very gradually be encouraged to move on their tummies in a circle using their arms and legs to reach a desired object close by. The key is to present several different objects to keep the infant's interest. Often this approach is more satisfying for the infant and a more effective means of gaining head control than using a wedge under the chest. The wedge can lock the infant into the position, making it more difficult to lift the head and turn over. Although the wedge does not promote active movement, it does keep the infant in the prone position. The amount of time spent in prone depends primarily on the infant's tolerance.

Since the goal of devices and equipment is to provide the opportunity for safe movement with optimal body alignment, "locking" babies into positioning devices in supine, sidelying, and prone so that they cannot move independently must be done with caution. Short periods in static positions permit the caregiver to interact with the child and encourage repetition of reaching and looking. On the other hand, leaving a little flexibility so that infants can explore their space in these positions is also recommended. If prone experiences during waking periods are positive and the infant is moved out of this position before becoming frantic, it is easier to build up tolerance. However, allowing infants to sleep in prone is not a good idea. Always follow the recommendations of your family physician regarding the amount of time your baby spends lying on the tummy.

Adaptation of Devices and Equipment for Infants

Commercially available types of baby equipment such as infant seats, swings, highchairs, and bath supports are routinely used by parents of children with osteogenesis imperfecta. However, fit and alignment are important. Since these items are usually designed from a one-size-fits-all perspective; they can be too big for children with osteogenesis imperfecta, who may be quite small for their age. Families must be ready to modify or adapt equipment if necessary, and occupational or physical therapists can be very helpful in this process. When choosing commercial equipment and devices for infants, families must be careful to select models that provide head support and allow easy access. It is important to avoid leaving the baby in the same position in any device for an extended period.

Car seats

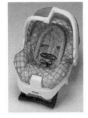

Figure 4. An infant car seat.

Small babies with osteogenesis imperfecta are best transported in an infant car seat (Figure 4) rather than in the larger type meant for children up to 7 years old. The already mentioned *head-hugger,* a simple support pillow to position the baby's head in midline, is strongly recommended. Small rolls can be placed beside the legs if external rotation and abduction of the hips is a big problem. The Dream Ride car bed by Cosco is a crash-tested car seat recommended for very low birth-weight babies (Figure 5). This piece of equipment can be used with the baby in supine or later in a semi-reclined position.

Parents are discouraged from adding layers of foam between the plastic base of car seat and the padded cover. Foam compresses

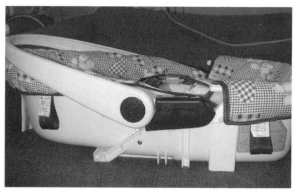

Figure 5. A car bed.

too easily in case of impact and the fit of the straps will not be accurate. Folded sheets or receiving blankets are suggested instead, if the child's caretakers insist on extra softness. Parents are reminded that the safest place in a vehicle is the back seat. Stopping every 30 to 60 minutes and removing the baby from the car seat during a long trip is strongly recommended.

Once a baby weighs more than 20 pounds, a *full-sized car seat* is necessary. The best choices are models with low sides, a five-point harness, wide straps, and no flip-down bar. These models adapt well to any modifications needed in case of lower extremity fracture. Any car seat should be used in the rear-facing position for as long as the weight limit requires.

If a child weighing between 20 and 40 pounds requires a spica brace or cast, the Spelcast car seat by Snug Seat can be a useful option (Figure 6). This crash-tested car seat was designed for children with congenital hip problems but can be used for any child in a hip spica cast. Easter Seals or local medical centers generally loan these specialized car seats to families because they are very expensive to purchase for temporary use. Snug Seat discontinued Spelcast production in 2004 in favor of a newly designed car seat by Britax.

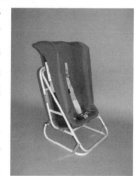

Figure 6. A Spelcast car seat.

The *stroller* is a critical piece of equipment for any family. It is also the piece of equipment used the longest, so paying more for good quality is probably the most economical strategy. Everyone needs a model that is sturdy yet light and easy to fold. Some families find it convenient to also have a very light, foldable model for travel. The umbrella stroller model with firm upholstery is suggested.

Additional stroller features recommended for children with osteogenesis imperfecta:
• Adjustable positions, allowing placement of the infant from completely reclined to semireclined to upright sitting
• A removable bar or no bar in front to allow easy entry and exit
• Good suspension in all four wheels and swivel wheels for a smooth ride

Baby jumpers are often a favorite piece of equipment used by parents to stimulate and pacify babies. However, infants with osteogenesis imperfecta are at risk in jumpers because of the fragility of their long bones, particularly the femora, or thigh bones. Baby jumpers are not recommended, and the use of baby walkers can also be risky if the child catches one leg or falls in the walker.

Devices and Equipment That Can Help Promote Sitting Balance

Reclined infant seats or bouncers are very common and are usually the first devices used to place the infant in a semisitting position. Most models provide a semireclined position (45 to 60 degrees of incline). The infant car seat carrier is also used in the home as a first seat, as it provides a similar angle of recline for the young infant. Adding mobiles or toy bars at 4 to 5 months of age is wonderful for encouraging active reaching and grasping.

Baby swings are very popular with families of new babies because of their effectiveness in soothing the cranky infant. The best models are those with a recline or tilt feature for the young infant with emerging head control. The commercial sleep positioners mentioned above help cradle the infant into a symmetrical position while in the swing. However, it is important that very young infants who do not have head and trunk control do not spend more than a few minutes swinging if good postural alignment cannot be maintained in the device.

The *boppy pillow*, a soft, crescent-shaped piece of upholstered foam sometimes referred to as a nursing pillow, is the ideal piece of equipment to promote gentle progression toward more independent sitting (Figure 7). It can be used in a stroller or high-chair or simply as support when playing on the floor.

Corner seats can be useful for increasing sitting endurance once babies have developed some head and trunk control. They are available in rubber and vinyl from durable medical equipment vendors or are made from wood and plastic in a workshop. Once again, they should be used for short periods, 15 to 30 minutes, to avoid widely abducted and externally rotated hips. The child should be removed from the seat when fatigued or unable to sit symmetrically.

Another simple piece of equipment used to promote sitting is the circular bath support with suction cups (Figure 8). This can be used outside the tub when the baby has achieved some static balance but still needs minimal support. Again, however, the infant's posture in this device should be carefully monitored to promote symmetrical weight-bearing over the spine, rather than having the infant sway or weave in the seat with a very lax or unstable spine.

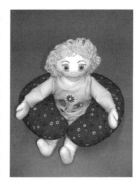

Figure 7. A boppy pillow.

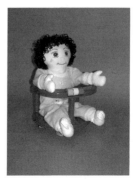

Figure 8. A bath support.

Adaptive or custom seating

For children who are very fragile and slow to achieve milestones, adaptive seating may be necessary. The different options depend on the resources available in each community. One option is customized seating devices made to measure for the child using either ABS plastic and foam or wood and foam. Another option is commercial therapeutic seating, such as the Kid Kart and the Kimba, available in several sizes from durable medical equipment suppliers (see the list at the end of this chapter and Chapter 8 for specific vendors). Both options help babies with osteogenesis imperfecta acquire the sitting position gradually and sitting balance safely. In both cases these seats should be made to closely fit the smaller dimensions of the baby with osteogenesis imperfecta. Accurate fit provides good support and is useful to minimize the potential for deformity of the spine and ribs.

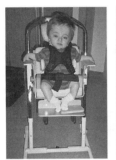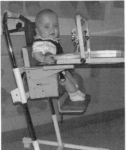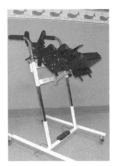

Figure 9. Custom seating options.

Ideally these seats should have an adjustable seat-back angle and tilt-in-space mechanism so the baby can be brought to the upright position gradually (Figure 9). Placing the seating system on a wheeled base (either a stroller or a highchair) is a convenient and practical solution for families.

Important accessories for custom seats include:
• Removable headrests (once head control is achieved)
• Footrests allowing 90 degree knee and ankle flexion angles
• Trays
• Removable cotton slipcovers to absorb the increased perspiration of babies with osteogenesis imperfecta

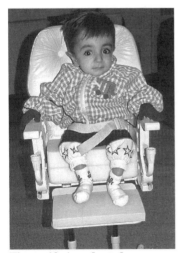

Figure 10. An adapted highchair.

Other ideas that work well with seating devices to stimulate fine motor and play development are an outrigger on the tray for hanging toys and a small wedge-on tray for propping books.

Some babies with osteogenesis imperfecta demonstrate fairly good motor development and may be ready to use a regular highchair (Figure 10). One problem, however, is that the commercial highchairs are deep and wide. Babies with osteogenesis imperfecta, who are usually of smaller stature, sit in the standard highchair with legs extended, but in an abducted, externally rotated position.

Regular highchairs are acceptable, but it is strongly recommended that the seat depth be decreased by adding foam or a blanket cushion to the back. A footrest at the appropriate height is necessary as well, so that the hips, knees, and ankles are flexed to 90 degrees and the feet are supported.

Devices and Equipment to Help Achieve Standing

The nonring infant walkers known as exersaucers (Figure 11) can be used to introduce infants to early foot weight-bearing and activation of the hip muscles (adductors) to bring the legs together. They also encourage the sit-to-stand transition. It is essential that the seat of such a device be positioned so the child is in a 90-degree sitting position. If positioned too high, the device

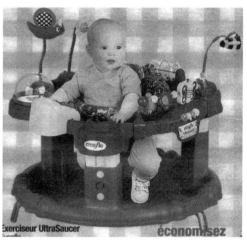

Figure 11. An exersaucer.

fosters an inappropriate weight-bearing position, possibly increasing the risk for fracture and increased bowing of the femora. The treating physician should be consulted about such a device to avoid these potential problems.

It is important to note that commercial ring walkers on wheels are not appropriate for infants, especially those with osteogenesis imperfecta, as babies can accidentally fall on stairs or tip over with these devices. For this reason, they are no longer available in Canada or the United States except at yard sales.

Toddlers with osteogenesis imperfecta who have never walked with or without walking aids can be gradually introduced to the vertical position by means of a tilt table (Figure 12), a supine stander, or a prone stander. This should be done very gradually so children are comfortable in the device and attain standing at their own pace. Ensure sufficient lateral support by adding rolls. Tilt tables are available in most physical therapy departments. Check the January 1973 issue of the *Journal of the American Physical Therapy Association* for how to make an easy, inexpensive tilt table for toddlers.

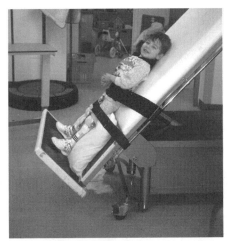

Figure 12. A tilt table.

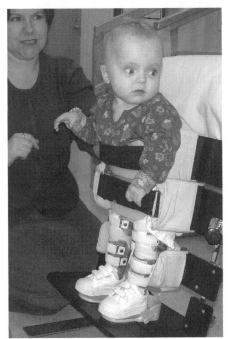

Figure 13. A supine stander.

Supine standers are available in various sizes through rehabilitation equipment companies. A physical therapist can work with the vendor to help determine the correct size for your child. Children who have recently had femoral or tibial roddings but never walked prior to surgery can start standing with or without braces on the tilt table or supine stander beginning at a 15- to 30-degree angle and progressing gradually until they are able to stand for 30 to 40 minutes at an angle of 75 degrees. It is important to remember to securely fasten the child onto the tilt table or supine stander so the child feels secure and accidents can be averted.

Prone standers, on which the child faces the device, are readily available in most physical therapy departments and schools. They are, however, not comfortable for children who have prominent and fragile ribcages or weak head and trunk control. Thus, a prone stander should not be the first stander chosen. In addition, many prone standers do not offer the option of bringing the child up gradually, as does a supine stander (Figure 13). It is crucial to be able to remove the child from the stander easily and quickly if a problem occurs. Some standers offer the option of being used as prone or supine standers.

The Totstander by Leckey is a new stander from Ireland that can be useful for young children with osteogenesis imperfecta (Figure 14). It is extremely light-weight, adjustable, and portable. Children should be gradually introduced to such a device, starting with 15 minutes and progressing to a maximum of 45 minutes. As with all other devices that touch the skin, any redness on the skin should not persist beyond a maximum of 15 minutes once out of the stander.

Devices and Equipment to Help Achieve Mobility and Ambulation

Every child with osteogenesis imperfecta is unique when it comes to ambulation or walking. The spectrum of severity inherent in this condition and the new treatments available make it difficult to predict who will walk, when walking will begin, what devices might be needed in order to walk, and with what degree of endurance.

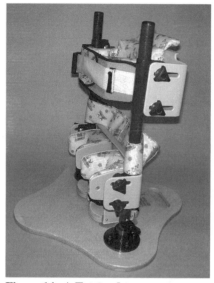

Figure 14. A Totstander.

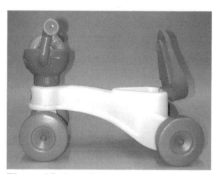

Figure 15. A push toy.

Wheeled seated push toys (Figure 15) are a great idea for the child beginning to initiate independent mobility because they encourage the transition from sitting to standing. Children develop strength in their legs as they learn how to maneuver these wheeled toys. Children usually learn to propel themselves backwards before they learn to go forward. Look for a model that has a narrow seat so as to properly fit shorter legs.

Some models have extensions in the back to enable the child to walk while wheeling the toy. Although this is an excellent means of perfecting walking, it can be dangerous if the toy is too light. The child could fall forward. Various models have small compartments in the seat of the toy in which

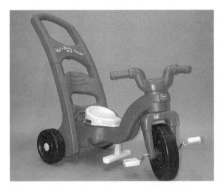

Figure 16. A three-in-one wheeled toy.

weights can be placed. A 5-pound weight is usually sufficient. A weighted kiddie shopping cart is also an alternative.

A variety of multipurpose versatile devices are on the commercial market for the infant who is gaining the skills necessary to walk. Fisher-Price has a three-in-one toy that can be converted from a rocking horse to a parent-propelled wheeled toy to a regular low-riding push toy or tricycle (Figure 16).

Most children with a moderate to severe form of osteogenesis imperfecta need some type of mobility device for long distances or outdoor walking and other activities in the early years. Many need these devices following fractures or surgery. Some families choose a manual wheelchair or other self-propelled device with a view to providing the child with independence. Some families choose a parent-propelled device such as a stroller for this period, trying to encourage walking as much as possible. Clearly there are pros and cons to both options and the decision is based on the individual needs and personality of the child and family. Our experience has been that the best plan is to make the variety of options match the multitude of situations of daily life.

Parent-propelled locomotor devices

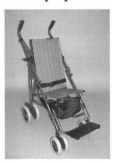

Figure 17. A stroller for larger children.

A good-quality stroller is a valid option for many older children because it is sized to fit those up to 5 years of age. Larger strollers built for children weighing up to 60 to 100 pounds (Figure 17) are the Major Buggy by Maclaren, the Cruiser by Convaid, and the Eco-Buggy by Otto Bock. Although these models fit the older child, they may be unsuitable because they are designed to meet the developmental needs of a younger child and may not suit an older child's personal image.

Self-propelled riding devices

Adapted tricycles (Figure 18) provide a safe method of mobility in which children diagnosed with osteogenesis imperfecta are able to keep up with their peers and strengthen their leg muscles at the same time. Children who require trunk support for balance are provided with a simple trunk support that can be attached to most commercially available tricycles. Pedal attachments can be added if needed.

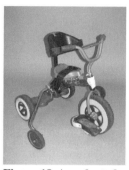

Figure 18. An adapted tricycle.

Regular tricycles are unstable and can turn over during turns because of their tripod design. However, a stabilizing bar with small wheels (a type of training wheels) can be added to ensure stability (Figure 19). Low-riding three-wheelers are preferred because they are closer to the ground, provide greater stability, promote self-propulsion with the feet on the ground, and allow independent transfers onto and off the vehicle.

Nontippable three-wheelers (low riding tricycles) can be useful alternatives to wheelchairs at home or at school. Riding vehicles are common play equipment for all children and easily accepted by parents. In some countries, three-wheelers of various sizes and models are the mobility devices of choice. Children are typically most functional when they incorporate a variety of devices and pieces of therapeutic equipment into their daily lives.

Self-propelled locomotor devices (manual wheelchairs)

Around age 2 it is important to start thinking about independent mobility. Children with osteogenesis imperfecta may be scooting or crawling or perhaps using a walker, but they also need an appropriate mobility device to be independent and at the same height as their peers. A wheelchair can be considered at this time. Less involved children may need the wheelchair only after a fracture, at school for safety reasons, or for long distances or outdoors. More involved children use wheelchairs indoors and outdoors. The wheelchair prescription can be challenging because of the small stature of children with osteogenesis imperfecta.

Considerations that can help in wheelchair selection:

• The narrowest possible width facilitates access to wheels for independent

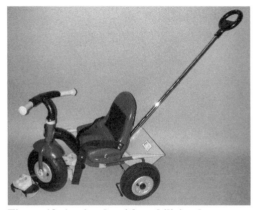

Figure 19. A tricycle with stabilizing bar.

propulsion
- Camber wheels increase wheelchair stability
- Seat depth for the crossbars and seat are specific to the child, but some parents prefer to order the chassis approximately 4 inches longer to allow the footrests to act as bumpers
- Seat-to-floor height should be adjusted according to the child's and parent's needs
- Rear wheel size should provide the optimal position for the child's arms to access the wheels for propulsion
- Brake extensions allow independent operation for children with short arms
- For older, especially heavy children, swing-away footrests can make standing transfers easier, but they add more weight to propel for younger, lighter children and are easily lost
- Removable leg supports for support in case of fracture may be indicated for older children

Frequently clinicians and vendors order wheelchairs somewhat larger than needed to anticipate growth. This practice is strongly discouraged for children with osteogenesis imperfecta as it contributes to improper positioning and makes it more difficult for the child to propel the added unnecessary weight. Every effort should be made to obtain as light a chair as is reasonable for a specific child's needs.

Adolescents may want to consider a rigid-frame wheelchair (Figure 20). This model of wheelchair, although slightly more awkward to store and fold, is more efficient for propulsion and turning. These features are critical for mobility in the community and with peers. Although a rigid-frame wheelchair can also be easier for a younger child to propel, it can be more costly to enlarge. Manual propulsion of wheelchairs strengthens the arms and expends calories. If the child has radial head dislocation, caution about arm position with respect to wheel rim is essential. Backpacks, either on the back of the chair or under the seat for rigid-frame models, are essential for the school years.

Power wheelchairs

Children with extremely weak, bowed upper extremities, extremely short stature, reduced pulmonary function, and limited independent mobility may need a power wheelchair (Figure 21) in order to experience a functional means of moving around outside the home. In rare instances, power tilt can be indicated if the child is unable to tolerate upright sitting for an extended period. To the extent possible, it is important to encourage every child to develop and experience some form of independent locomotion, be it rolling, commando crawling, or scooting in addition to power mobility. In general, the child using a power chair is not a candidate for a manual wheelchair. Families are encouraged to consider selecting power mobility as the main mobility when it is the only means by which the child can move around outdoors independently.

Invacare and Sunrise Medical both have pediatric power wheelchairs with smaller bases and seat components for the smaller stature. Standard joystick control is used.

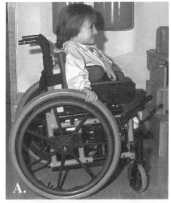

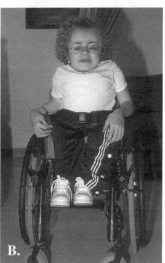

Figure 20. A rigid-frame wheelchair, side and front views.

Power chairs on which the seat goes up and down and reclines are an option that allows adjustability of seat height. This option is particularly indicated for the child with severe fragility or weakness because it can provide the ability to get into and out of the chair and onto the floor independently for children who would otherwise be dependent for transfers. With this device many surfaces can be accessed, including the floor from the lowest seat position. The Permobil chair and the Jazzy offer a seat elevator with a range going as low as floor level (Figure 22). Permobil also has an excellent model

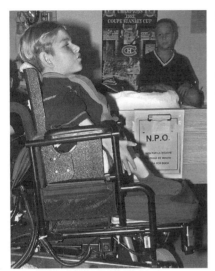

Figure 21. A power wheelchair.

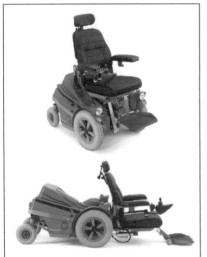

Figure 22. A power wheelchair with a hi-low seat.

for tiny children called the Koala.

Walkers

Children start walking or ambulating with the assistance of walkers and in some cases long leg braces as discussed in Chapter 2. Many types of walking aids are available, but consultation with the treating physical therapist is necessary to determine the appropriate device based on the needs of the child.

Considerations when deciding on appropriate walking aids include:

- Height, width, and weight of the child
- Posture of the child when standing
- Child's leg and arm strength
- Standing balance the child has achieved
- Standing balance when walking with such a device
- Surface on which the child will walk (floor, carpet, outdoors)
- Child's endurance for walking

When toddlers and older children begin to walk for the first time, their tendency is to protect themselves from a fall by reaching forward with their hands. A stable two-wheeled *forward rollator walker* (Figure 23) is usually the walker of choice for children with osteogenesis imperfecta who are beginning to walk. The Tyke aluminum infant walker by Guardian has proved successful with this population of children. The advantage of the two-wheeled walker is that the rubber tips located in the back limit backward movement and provide greater stability when the child stands up by pressing down on the hand grips of the device.

Several companies manufacture walkers made of lightweight aluminum that can be used as both forward and reverse rollators. Once the child has become accustomed to the forward rollator (walker), the wheels can be reversed and the walker then is transformed into a reverse walker, which promotes erect standing when walking.

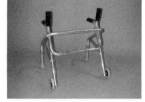

Figure 23. A forward rollator walker.

The *strider walker* is a lightweight rollator that is reversible and available in several sizes. The advantage of this type of walker is the variety of positions possible with use of the handgrips. This accommodates the forearm deformities sometimes seen in children with osteogenesis imperfecta. However, it must be noted that the strider can be less stable when used in the reverse mode. Caution must be taken when teaching a child how to use such a walking aid, and adequate supervision is crucial until the child is completely proficient. It is also recommended to remove all scatter rugs because walkers can get caught in them and tip over.

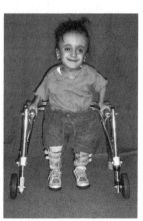

Figure 24. A posture control walker.

The Kaye *posture control walker* (Figure 24) can also be used in the forward or reverse modes. This walker is somewhat heavier than the strider but is extremely stable, especially in the reverse mode.

For the older child accustomed to the two-wheeled reverse model but who requires a walker for balance only, the Kaye *four-wheeled walker* with swivel front wheels has proved successful (Figure 25). Another option with the Kaye reverse walker is a seat that enables children with osteogenesis imperfecta to rest as they improve their endurance for walking.

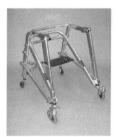

Figure 25. A four-wheeled walker.

The older child may require a sturdier *forward four-wheeled rollator* (Figure 26), which still provides ease of maneuverability. Some models have seats with or without back supports and shopping baskets. In addition, the

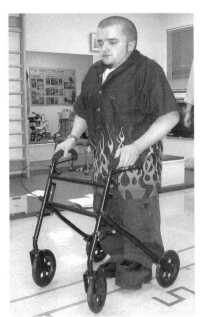

Figure 26. A forward four-wheeled rollator walker.

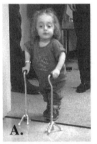 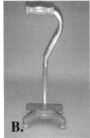

A.   B.

Figure 27. Quadripod canes.

large 8-inch wheels are ideal for absorbing the shock of bumpy terrain. Bicycle handle-type brakes often come with these rollators.

Some children who have deformities of their arms require adjustable forearm supports. For these children, choose a model, and size, that properly supports the forearms.

Canes and crutches

Some children with osteogenesis imperfecta progress from walkers to lightweight aluminum quadripod canes or crutches. Small-sized canes are not available, but it is possible to take a small adult size and cut the cane. Depending on the child, these canes can be preferable to forearm cuff (Lofstrand) crutches, as the children are less likely to lean forward on the quad canes than on the crutches. Lofstrand crutches can be problematic for children with a history of upper extremity fractures or radial head dislocations. They can be appropriate for children who do not yet have the balance to walk with the quad canes or if they prefer them to canes. If using Lofstrand crutches, make sure that the cuff openings are large enough for the arms to come out if the child falls. In addition, extra large crutch tips add to the stability of the device.

When a perfect fit cannot be obtained, rehabilitation and orthotic device companies can fabricate or adapt commercially available devices to meet the needs of the child. Figure 27 shows two examples.

Children with osteogenesis imperfecta seldom like to use axillary crutches, and the crutches promote poor alignment of the shoulders and back. In addition, some children do not transition through crutches to achieve independent walking because they feel insecure with them. Instead, these children often begin to walk among pieces of furniture at home without the walking aid and eventually graduate from using the walking aid to walking without any gait device.

Bracing and orthotic devices

Children with osteogenesis imperfecta have low bone mineral density and can have decreased bone mass, muscle weakness of the hips and legs, and contractures that interfere with the ability to maintain upright posture without external support. Bracing the legs can provide needed limb support, maintain a functional position, or promote motion of a body part. Bivalve or "clam shell" bracing can be used as a light-weight replacement for a plaster cast following surgery or fracture.

Upright activity requires muscular effort, bone loading, and proprioceptive input (a sense of where the leg has been placed that requires sensation and position awareness). Strengthening, increased bone mineral density, and improved balance often result from upright activity.

Research has demonstrated that maintaining and increasing muscle mass through activity increases bone mineral density and thus strengthens the bones. Ultimately the level of function is increased when braces are used appropriately.

Children with significant ligamentous laxity can benefit from bracing to maintain proper alignment of the joints and to improve mechanical efficiency by stabilizing the joints. This is especially true in the foot and ankle region, but bracing also can be successfully used in some cases of knee laxity.

Long leg braces with a pelvic band can be prescribed for young children who have demonstrated the gross motor ability to kneel and are starting to pull to the standing position against furniture. These children have acquired the necessary gross motor skills and desire to walk. Some centers order these braces to help accomplish walking in children who are not yet able to kneel and pull up to stand because of hip and knee weakness.

These braces, or hip-knee-ankle-foot orthoses, are also known as HKAFOs (Figure 28). They have drop-lock joints at the hips and knees as well as movable ankle and foot sections. Single uprights are used for children who weigh less than 25 pounds and double uprights are used for children who

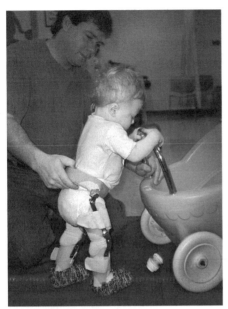

Figure 28. Walking with hip-knee-ankle-foot orthoses, or HKAFOs.

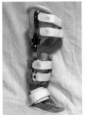

Figure 30. An ankle-foot orthosis, or AFO.

Figure 29. A knee-ankle-foot orthosis, or KAFO.

weigh more. Articulated orthoses are appropriate for standing and walking, but are not needed for children while sitting. These braces must be combined with an exercise program for the legs to counteract disuse atrophy, which can result from bracing without exercise.

Long leg braces without the pelvic band, known as knee-ankle-foot orthoses, or KAFOs, can be used to address a valgus alignment (an L shape) at the knees (Figure 29). For this situation, a solid ankle joint provides the best control.

Ankle-foot orthoses, or AFOs, can be prescribed to provide stability, better alignment of the foot and ankle, and improved gait efficiency for the tibia and foot (Figure 30).

It is very important that the braces be put on the child's legs very carefully to avoid fractures. Always place the child's leg into the brace without twisting the foot or knee. Attach the ankle strap before securing the other straps. If the skin is red for more than 15 minutes after removal of the brace, it is not fitting properly or it was not put on correctly.

For the infant with significant ligamentous laxity who is learning to stand and cruise around furniture but does not require full leg bracing, an in-shoe orthotic device (Figure 31) can provide the midfoot support necessary for gross motor development and balance during this critical phase. These orthotic devices include off-the-shelf soft components that are available commercially.

There are a variety of options for children and adolescents with osteogenesis imperfecta regarding the management of foot discomfort that can occur especially after prolonged walking or any walking on uneven terrain. Although a custom-made shoe is rarely warranted, a well-made shoe is important for comfort. An athletic shoe with a soft upper section, a firm heel cup, a flexible sole that is wide at the heel, and a well-developed arch support provides the amount of contact and comfort required. In addition, a light shoe versus a heavy shoe enables the child to walk longer distances without fatigue or discomfort. A high-top shoe can provide additional ankle support for those who do not have severe alignment problems at the ankle.

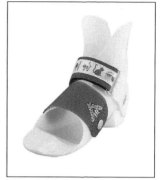

Figure 31. An in-shoe orthotic device.

For youngsters with severe flat feet or markedly pronated feet (Figure 32A), custom-made arch supports or heel cups (called UCBLs, for University of California Biomedical Laboratories) or above-the-ankle devices (called SMOs, for supramalleolar orthotics) that control the heel and foot are often prescribed. The recommended custom-made arch supports should be made of high- and/or low-density foam with polymer thermoplastics (Figure 32B).

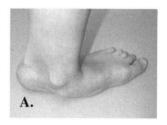

A.

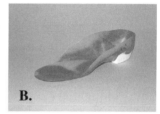

B.

Figure 32. A custom-made arch support for a flat or pronated foot.

Fitting an AFO into a regular athletic shoe can be challenging. First, try removing the foam liner in the regular shoe, which adds a depth of one-fourth inch to the shoe. If this additional space is insufficient, purchase wider shoes to accommodate the braces. Longer shoes can cause tripping. Alternatively, orthotic device companies stock "deep shoes" made especially to accommodate braces. Always try the brace in the shoe prior to purchase.

Miscellaneous braces and splints

Many commercial splints or braces are used for fracture management in osteogenesis imperfecta. Often a heavy cast is removed after an initial period

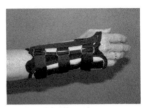

Figure 33. A wrist cock-up brace.

of immobilization and a light-weight, simple brace is provided that gives additional immobilization but is easier to remove for bathing and physical therapy.

Some children with osteogenesis imperfecta experience upper extremity orthopedic problems such as drop wrist and swan neck deformity of fingers. Braces commonly used for these conditions include the wrist cock-up brace, which keeps the wrist up and so allows easier finger movement (Figure 33). Ring splints are also used with swan neck deformities. These are stainless steel, silver, or gold finger rings whose figure-eight design stabilizes and prevents hyperextension.

Postsurgical bracing

Children with osteogenesis imperfecta who can pull up to standing position but who have had repeated leg fractures and significant femoral and/or tibial bowing usually undergo some form of intramedullary rodding. Telescoping rods are intended to elongate within the bone as the child grows. Occasionally nontelescoping rods are used for the femur. They can also be used for the tibia

Figure 34. An articulating AFO.

because of the difficulty of inserting telescoping rods into the ankle joint. Thus, tibial rods usually do not elongate within the bone. The tibia may continue to grow beyond the limits of the rod and can deform.

Some orthopedic surgeons prescribe HKAFOs with solid ankle joints 3 weeks after femoral and tibial roddings as an early replacement for plaster casts. When the thigh muscles (quadriceps) are strong enough to control the extension of the knee, the thigh sections are removed, creating a solid AFO. Within a few months, the solid AFOs are replaced with moveable, articulating AFOs (Figure 34) to permit free motion of the ankles and strengthening of the calf muscles. These muscles allow the child to rise onto the toes and permit a more fluid walking pattern.

Devices and Equipment to Help Achieve Independence in Activities of Daily Living

Adaptive devices are important if the child with osteogenesis imperfecta is to achieve full autonomy in the activities of daily living. Simple, common-sense solutions to daily challenges, as described below, often bridge the gap between dependence and independence. Grab bars, armrests, mats, and other devices provide an atmosphere of safety that is crucial for teaching and learning self-care and transfer tasks. It is worthwhile to note that involvement in self-care is an excellent opportunity to initiate and foster independence.

Often parents do more than necessary out of concern for fractures, for the sake of saving time, or merely out of habit. Therapists can show parents and children how to take a self-care activity and break it down into small, manageable components. For example, the child can start with putting the toothpaste on the toothbrush or buttoning up after the shirt is put on. Participation, no matter how small, promotes self-confidence and motivates the child to be more independent.

Getting on the toilet

A child-sized potty seat secured to the floor or a custom-made commode is an option for the child unable to transfer to a regular toilet. For children who can transfer, a regular toilet can be made more accessible. Some devices that are helpful for getting on and off the toilet are listed below.

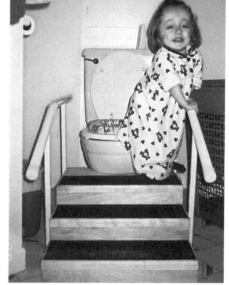

- A set of steps with handrails (Figure 35), a long wedge, or a small bench
- Grab bars, standard wall-mounted or flip-up style, which are very useful for ensuring safe standing or sliding transfer

Figure 35. Steps with handrails.

- A raised toilet seat (Figure 36) securely locked onto a regular toilet, which facilitates a sliding wheelchair transfer

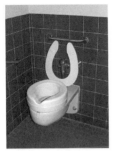

Figure 36. A lock-on raised seat.

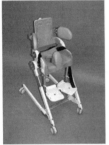

Figure 37. An adaptive toilet seat.

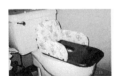

Figure 38. A padded reducer ring.

Sitting on the toilet

Some children with osteogenesis imperfecta require equipment for extra support in sitting. They need to feel secure to free one hand for hygiene while sitting on the more precarious surface. Some suggestions are listed below.

• Several vendors distribute toilet seats like the Flamingo by Snug Seat that are placed over the regular toilet and offer back, trunk, and arm support (Figure 37)

• A padded reducer ring, available at most hardware and baby stores, provides a larger sitting surface while reducing the opening (Figure 38)

• Some families prefer to fabricate their own toilet seat to match their child's particular needs; for example, the adaptive seat may need to also support fragile extended legs

Hygiene

Children with short, bowed, or fragile upper extremities can have difficulty with the hygienic aspect of toileting. The devices listed below can increase autonomy.

• A male or female urinal and bedpan for use on the bed surface if the child can manage only a rolling or sliding transfer on the same level

• A toilet aid made of Plexiglas or ABS plastic that is 6 inches long and angled with a slit for toilet paper to assist in reaching the perineal area (Figure 39)

• A dressing stick to assist with pulling pants up and down

• Wet-Ones or other disposable moist

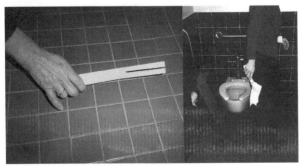

Figure 39. A toilet aid.

towlettes to ease wiping
- Commercial hygiene sprays, such as Lubidet (see Table 1)

Bathing

Getting into the bath or shower. Understandably, this skill is often difficult to attain because the environment is inherently slippery. Parents are often over-protective and tend to help with this daily task for a long period. However, with caution, practice, and the appropriate equipment, children with osteogenesis imperfecta can learn to be independent at bath time. Suggestions regarding equipment include:

- Steps
- A platform linking the toilet and bath ledge
- A plastic two-step stool on the outside of the tub and a one-step stool inside the tub to facilitate sitting entry
- A transfer tub seat (Figure 40)
- A power bath lift
- A roll-in shower chair
- Grab bars

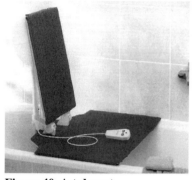

Figure 40. A tub seat.

Sitting or standing in the bath or shower. Once in the bathtub or shower, adaptive devices can promote safety and increase independence. Some examples include a:

- Bath trunk support
- Reclined bath seat
- Commercial bath ring
- Shower or bath bench/chair (Figure 41)
- Rubber bathmat
- Hand-held shower source

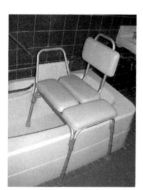

Figure 41. A bench/
chair for bathtub or
shower.

Three types of bath supports for use in the tub are available. One is the built-in wedge of the plastic baby bath. Another is the simple wire wedge covered in terry cloth used in conjunction with the baby bath. The third type is the foam bath insert, which positions and protects the infant. Older children can use the plastic booster seat intended for the kitchen as a bath seat. The seat, back, and armrests provide support when it is placed inside the tub.

The bath. A long-handled bath sponge can facilitate independence while bathing, as can levered handles on sink taps, and a reacher to access bath faucets.

Dressing and grooming

Children with osteogenesis imperfecta usually master the tasks of dressing and grooming. However, they may take longer to acquire these skills. Children with short and bowed upper extremities do have more difficulty and may need technical aids and adapted equipment to complete the task quickly and be independent. These aids include:
- Dressing sticks of appropriate length to reach the lower extremities
- Reachers
- Lower clothes rods in closets
- A long-handled hairbrush
- Bureaus and counters at appropriate height
- Front-opening garments, which can be easier to don than garments that pull on over the head

Accessibility

When a wheelchair, power or manual, is the main mobility device, families need to address the issue of accessibility of the home and of the vehicle used to transport the child. Families may choose less expensive, temporary solutions initially, then decide on more permanent long-term adaptations. Several generic options from the huge range of available adaptations are listed below in order of expense. It is strongly recommended to consult therapists and companies with specific expertise in adapting homes and vehicles.

The home
- Wood or concrete entry ramps; the grade should be 1:12 for self-propulsion or 1:8 for caregiver-provided propulsion
- Outdoor elevator platforms; generally used when the entrance is more

than 3 feet from the ground
- Indoor elevators, allowing access to basement or upper floor levels
- Bathroom access for the wheelchair

The vehicle
- Folding or telescoping ramps; available in one flat piece or as two single rails
- A tie-down system to secure the wheelchair inside the vehicle (required when someone is being transported in a wheelchair)
- A posterior head support on the wheelchair for use during transport
- A powered platform lift and raised roof
- A lowered floor with a kneeling mechanism and powered ramp
- Adaptation of the steering and/or braking mechanism for drivers

Devices for Strengthening

Children and adults diagnosed with osteogenesis imperfecta can participate in a wide range of interesting and safe strengthening programs designed to increase endurance as well as strength. Swimming, other recreational activities, and adapted sports are good examples discussed in Chapters 5 and 6. Safe methods of muscle strengthening include weight-bearing using the standing and walking devices described above. Seat push-ups from a chair, wheelchair, or stool are also safe and helpful (Figure 42). The ultimate purpose of these activities is to enhance the performance of the child, adolescent, and adult.

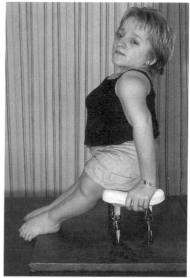

Figure 42. Seat push-ups build strength, but may not be indicated when the arms are bowed.

Exercise with light free weights
An individual program using weights can be appropriate for some children and adults with osteogenesis imperfecta and can be established for a specific

child, adolescent, or adult by the treating physical therapist. Before the use of resistive devices such as light free weights is considered, the person must be able to move the arms and legs and head and trunk through space without assistance. Since one's own weight can also be used as a resistance force, great caution is indicated before using external weights for resistance, especially if there is bowing of the bones. Since ligamentous laxity is present in many people with osteogenesis imperfecta, external weight used for resistance can put additional strain on joints that are already loose. Finally, weight applied at the end of the arm or leg (distally), around the wrist or ankle, can provide sufficient stress to fracture the bone.

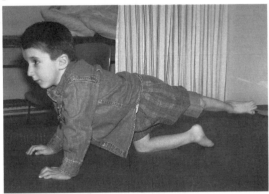

Figure 43. Light-resistance exercise.

Light resistance using external weights can be appropriate for strengthening for some children with osteogenesis imperfecta, particularly adolescents and adults. Weights in increments of one-fourth pound are placed proximally, above the bowing of the bone (Figure 43). A weight as light as half a tube of toothpaste can be used to strengthen the shoulder and elbow muscles, and can provide novelty and a sense of accomplishment for children, and parents, who need a change of pace.

Conclusion

Active movement in a safe environment is an essential concept for people with osteogenesis imperfecta to achieve optimal function. As the child progresses through the various stages of motor development and gradually gains independence, the use of appropriate devices and pieces of equipment can be the crucial element in achieving functional independence. Each person's situation, and potential, is unique and changes frequently with accomplishment and maturity. Therefore, individual children, adults, and families require different things at different times. We hope the suggestions and guidelines in this chapter will be of assistance in selecting these items.

Table 1. A Selected List of Devices, Equipment, and Vendors.

The devices mentioned are for illustration only; inclusion does not imply endorsement. Chapter 8 also lists many equipment resources.

Generic Product	Examples of Specific Brands	Examples of Specific Companies
Baby equipment by various manufacturers, including sleep positioners, head supports, pads, toys	1-2-3 Discovery Lane Playmat	**Dreamtime Baby** 3517 Schaefer Street Culver City, CA 90232 1-866-DRM-TIME www.dreamtimebaby.com
		Baby Abby 1157 S. Cherokee Street Denver, CO 80223 1-800-972-7357 www.babyabby.com
Soft baby carriers, exercise aids, toys	Snugli ExerSaucer	**Evenflo Company** 1801 Commerce Drive Piqua, OH 45356 1-800-233-5921 www.evenflo.com www.snugli.com
Boppy pillows	Boppy	**Boppy** 602 Park Point Drive (Suite 150) Golden, CO 80401 1-888-77B-OPPY www.boppy.com
Car beds, car seats, strollers	Dream Ride	**Cosco** 2525 State Street Columbus, IN 47201 1-800-544-1108 www.coscojuvenile.com
Car seats, toilet and bath seats (pediatric)	Flamingo Wallaby Infant Seat Britax Car Seat (replacing Spelcast)	**Snug Seat** 10810 Independence Pointe Parkway Matthews, NC 28106 1-800-336-7684 www.snugseat.com
Strollers	Cruiser	**Convaid** P.O. Box 4209 Palos Verdes, CA 90274 1-888-266-8243 www.convaid.com
	Major Buggy	**Maclaren USA** 4 Testa Place South Norwalk, CT 06854 1-877-442-4622 www.maclarenbaby.com

Generic Product	Examples of Specific Brands	Examples of Specific Companies
Mobility systems, lifting devices	Eco-Buggy Kimba Pediatric Tilt-in-Space	**Otto Bock Health Care** 2 Carlson Parkway (Suite 100) Minneapolis, MN 55447-4467 1-800-328-4058 www.ottobockus.com
Bath seats, transfer tub seats, grab bars (basic adult), raised toilet seats	Sunmark Rubbermaid Dana Douglas	**Lumex Medical Supplies Plus** 29877 Telegraph Road (Suite 103) Southfield, MI 48034 1-800-794-8383 www.medicalsuppliesplus.com **Dana Douglas** P.O. Box 1324 Ogdensburg, NY 13669 613-723-6734 155 Colonnade Road (Unit 10) Nepean, Ontario K2E 7K1 1-800-267-3552 www.danadouglas.com
Bathing, mobility, toileting, exercise aids	Toilet Support Solutions	**Columbia Medical** P.O. Box 633 Pacific Palisades, CA 90272 1-800-454-5512 www.columbiamedical.com
Toilet commodes, reclined bath seats	Blue Wave	**Rifton Equipment** 359 Gibson Hill Road Chester, NY 10918-2321 1-800-777-4244 www.rifton.com
Personal hygiene products, toilet accessories	Lubidet	**Lubidet USA** **DesignCrew** 820 S. Monaco Parkway (Suite 353) Denver, CO 80224 1-800-582-4338 www.lubidet.com
Powered bath lifts	Aquatec Beluga	**Clark Health Care Products** 1003 International Drive Oakdale, PA 15071-9226 1-888-347-4537 www.clarkhealthcare.com **Dolomite Home** 50 Shields Court Markham, Ontario L3R 9T5 1-888-687-2390 www.dolomitehcp.com

Generic Product	Examples of Specific Brands	Examples of Specific Companies
Bath and shower mats, safety aids	Safti-Grip	**Rubbermaid Home Products Division** 3320 W. Market Street Fairlawn, OH 44333-3306 1-888-895-2110
Corner seats, walkers, wheelchairs, aids to daily living	Tumble Forms Guardian Strider	**Sammons Preston Rolyan–Canada** 755 Queensway East (Unit 27) Mississauga, Ontario L4Y 4C5 800-665-9200 www.sammonspreston.com
Wheelchair and stroller positioning systems and wheeled bases	Kid Kart Kid Kart Xpress Zippie Quickie	**Sunrise Medical** 7477 East Dry Creek Parkway Longmont, CO 80503 1-800-333-4000 www.sunrisemedical.com
Manual wheelchairs, power wheelchairs, hi-low power seats	Comet Action Storm Permobil Robo	**Invacare** One Invacare Way Elyria, OH 44035-4190 1-800-333-6900 570 Matheson Boulevard E (Unit 8) Mississauga, Ontario L4Z 4G4 1-800-668-5324 www.invacare.com
	Permobil Koala	**Permobil** 6961Eastgate Boulevard Lebanon, TN 37090 1-800-736-0925 www.permobilusa.com
	Jazzy	**Pride Mobility Products** 149 Winchendon Road Ashburnham, MA 01430 877-585-4041 www.jamesonmedical.com
Wheelchairs, sports wheelchairs	Colours in Motion	**Colours in Motion** 1591 S. Sinclair Street Anaheim, CA 92806 714-978-1440 www.colourswheelchair.com
Wheelchairs for sports, walkers, daily activity aids	Minova	**Etac Sverige AB** Customer Service, Box 203 SE–334 24 Anderstorp, Sweden +46-371-58-73-00 www.etac.net
Orthotics: long leg braces, short leg braces, ankle braces	HKAFOs, KAFOs, AFOs	**J. E. Hanger** 5545 St-Jacques Street West Montreal, Quebec H4A 2A3 514-489-8213

Generic Product	Examples of Specific Brands	Examples of Specific Companies
Shoe orthoses	Hotdog Pattibob	**Cascade DAFO** 1360 Sunset Avenue Ferndale, WA 98248 1-800-848-7332 www.dafo.com
Finger ring splints	Realignment Splint	**Digisplint** 476 Main Street South (Suite 9) Exeter, Ontario N0M 1S1 519-235-2981 www.digisplint.ca
Tilt tables, physical therapy equipment	Midland	**Cardon Rehabilitation Products** P.O. Box 237 Niagara Falls, NY 14304-0257 1-800-944-7868 38 A Buttermill Avenue Concord, Ontario L4K 3X3 905-761-7868 www.cardonrehab.com
Standers, seating and positioning devices	Totstander	**Leckey** (Distributed by **Sammons Preston**) 755 Queensway East (Unit 27) Mississauga, Ontario L4Y 4C5
Posture control walkers, forearm support walkers	Kaye Walker (various)	**Kaye Products** 535 Dimmocks Mill Road Hillsborough, NC 27278 1-800-685-5293 www.kayeproducts.com
Forearm crutches	Walk Easy Lofstrand	**Walk Easy** 601 N. Congress Avenue (Suite 204) Delray Beach, FL 33445-4627 1-800-441-2904 www.walkeasy.com
Quadripod canes, forearm crutches	Quad Lite Red Dot Quickfit Tyke	**Guardian Products** 4175 Guardian Street Simi Valley, CA 93063 1-800-255-5022
Wheeled toys, three-in-one toys	Fisher-Price Babygear	**Fisher-Price** Consumer Affairs 636 Girard Avenue East Aurora, NY 14052 1-800-432-5437 1-800-567-7724 (Canada) www-fisher-price.com

Generic Product	Examples of Specific Brands	Examples of Specific Companies
Learning and sports toys	Little Tike TotSports	**Little Tike Central** 2512-B Beech Street Valparaiso, IN 46383 1-866-311-8697 www.littletikecentral.com
Tricycles	Kettler	**Kettler International** P.O. Box 2747 Virginia Beach, VA 23450-2747 757-427-2400 www.kettlerusa.com

CHAPTER EIGHT

INFORMATION RESOURCES— WHAT'S OUT THERE?

A hard copy of virtual and other resources pertinent to people with osteogenesis imperfecta

Timothy J. Caruso, PT, MBA, MS

Goals:
- Explain how to judge the accuracy of medical information on the Internet
- Identify and describe sources of information related to osteogenesis imperfecta
- Identify and describe sources of adaptive equipment, adaptive sports, and funding resources related to managing osteogenesis imperfecta

Chapter Outline:
1. Information Credibility
2. Organizations and Other Web Resources
3. Support Services
4. Educational Materials
5. Resources for Devices and Adaptive Equipment
6. Funding Resources
7. Sports and Recreation
8. Appendixes
    A. *Information Credibility*
    B. *Devices and Adaptive Equipment*
    C. *Federally Funded National Organizations for People with Special Needs*

D. *Funding and Advocacy Groups*
E. *Magazines, Medical Journals, and Other Publications*
F. *Sports, Recreation, and Activity Camps*
G. *Travel Information and Driving Programs*
H *Quick Phone Number Reference List*
I. *Quick Web References*

1. Information Credibility

In opening the door to the information age for people with osteogenesis imperfecta and their families, it is important to clarify the concept of information credibility. Potentially thousands of information sources are available, including a number of organizations, Web pages, books, medical journals, commercial products and manufacturers. The Internet or "information highway" has transformed our ability to access information. No longer is it necessary to go to the library or to wait for tomorrow's newspaper or a radio or television broadcast. Information is available instantaneously in real time. The challenge is to identify what is relevant and credible and to do so in a timely fashion.

In this chapter many sources of information are discussed along with some potential pitfalls related to the Internet. The goal is to provide a few road signs to guide your Internet journey as an informed consumer. Please keep in mind that this is a small part of the big picture; an all-inclusive list would be impossible. Information credibility is an important issue. As has been observed about the Internet, bad information seems to have wider distribution and a longer shelf life than good information.

One big problem that has arisen from the tremendous growth of the Internet is that it is unmonitored as a whole. No one is keeping an eye on Internet content. Webmasters often copy information from one source to another without checking its accuracy. People can put what they wish on the Internet, and it may or may not be truthful, correct, accurate, fair, or legitimate. No matter where your research takes you, credibility and caution need to guide you. One large caution is to be truly mindful of the source of the information. Many sources are credible, reliable, and accurate. However, other sources of information are inaccurate, misleading, and just plain wrong. If the goal is to use information to make a life-changing decision, verifying the credibility, reliability, and accuracy of the information source is crucial. Webmasters can have ulterior motives; they can be con artists, or just plain ignorant. Interestingly enough, several recent publications have identified a number of errors on legitimate, scientific Web sites. Unintentional errors can still have a negative impact on someone's life. The importance of legitimate, correct information as it relates to one's health cannot be overstated.

Some medical Web sites are adopting rules and guidelines that address ethical issues as they relate to information sharing. One group that has taken the lead in this area is the Health on the Net Foundation, or HON (www.hon.ch). They have established a code of conduct for their site that nicely summarizes the criteria one should consider when viewing a Web site. Their eight-point code of conduct is as follows:

• *Authority.* Any medical or health advice provided and hosted on this site will be given only by medically trained and qualified professionals unless a clear statement is made that a piece of advice offered is from a non–medically qualified individual or organization.

• *Complementariness.* The information provided is designed to support, not replace, the relationship that exists between a patient or site visitor and his or her physician.

• *Confidentiality.* The confidential nature of data relating to individual patients and visitors to a medical or health Web site, including their identity, is respected. The site owners undertake to honor or exceed the legal requirements of medical and health information privacy that apply in the country and state where the Web site and mirror sites are located.

• *Attribution.* Where appropriate, information contained on this site will be supported by clear references to source data and, where possible, have specific HTML (the "hypertext markup language" of the World Wide Web) links to those data. The date when a clinical page was last modified will be clearly displayed (at the bottom of the page, for instance).

• *Justifiability.* Any claims relating to the benefits or performance of a specific treatment, commercial product, or service will be supported by appropriate, balanced evidence in this manner: Caution, care, buyer beware!

• *Transparency of ownership.* The designers of this Web site will seek to provide information in the clearest possible manner and provide contact addresses for visitors who seek further information or support. The

Webmaster will display his or her e-mail address clearly throughout the Web site.

- *Transparency of sponsorship.* Support for this Web site will be clearly identified, including the identities of commercial and noncommercial organizations that have contributed funding, services, or material for the site.
- *Honesty in advertising and editorial policy.* If advertising is a source of funding, it will be clearly stated. A brief description of the advertising policy adopted by the Web site owners will be displayed on the site. Advertising and other promotional material will be presented to viewers in a manner and context that facilitate differentiation between it and the original material created by the institution operating the site.

In spite of these efforts at information accuracy, most information sources are still a long way from the ideal situation in which users are able to register their specific needs, questions, concerns, and medications, for example, and have a custom-tailored response in return. Until such a Web site is available to consumers, the sites listed in this chapter will provide a good starting point for seeking information.

As a general rule, the Internet must be viewed as a source of additional information and not as the final word. Using the Internet must be an adjunct to, not the primary source of, decision-making. *Once information is gleaned from the Internet, it is vital to verify the information with your own health-care team.*

Another common problem is a Web site or search engine that redirects searches to other sites without letting the searcher know. This can occur numerous times during the course of a simple search; it is how most search engines operate, and it is not always readily apparent. Some search engines do this behind the scenes while others have a redirect notice on the bottom of the page. As you begin searching the Internet, keep this in mind when gathering information and be aware of the source. Numerous search engines exist, including All the Web, AltaVista, Google, HotBot, IXQuick, MetaCrawler, Metasearch, and Yahoo. Google has been identified by the *Wall Street Journal* as one of the top search engines on the World Wide Web.

Having a good search engine is invaluable; however, having a specific Web site tailored to meet some or all of your specific needs is even better. The Osteogenesis Imperfecta Foundation Web site (www.oif.org) is an ideal starting point for people with osteogenesis imperfecta. Another useful option might be to go to the Web site of the National Library of Medicine's MedlinePlus (www.medlineplus.gov) and input the information you have obtained about osteogenesis imperfecta and begin to look further. The advantage of utilizing a source such as the Osteogenesis Imperfecta Foundation or MedlinePlus is that it is screened information. Going to Google or another search engine can give you a larger quantity of information, but more caution has to be applied, as the Internet zone is completely unmonitored. See Appendix A for more on information credibility.

Start your successful Internet search by deciding what you are looking for. Begin with a general idea and then narrow it down as best you can. Is it a product or a service? If, for example, you type in the word "therapy," the result can be more than 1,000 sites. Being more specific by saying "physical therapy" or "occupational therapy" can narrow the number down to around 100. Plugging "osteogenesis imperfecta" into the MedlinePlus site yields more than 2,500 hits. A good way to keep track of helpful Web sites is to save them in the "favorites" section of your browser. Another way to keep them in order is to place them in folders with topic headings such as adaptive equipment, wheelchairs, sports, travel, etc.

We have listed numerous informational Web sites of interest in the Appendixes, but the list is certainly limited. With the rate at which things are changing on the Internet, many of these references may be long gone by the time this book is in your hands.

2. Organizations and Other Web Resources

Organizations that have Web sites can be good sources of reliable information. When using an organization Web site be aware that organizations gear their Web sites to different audiences—general users, adult patients, or medical practitioners.

The **Osteogenesis Imperfecta Foundation** (www.oif.org) is an organization dedicated to providing information about osteogenesis imperfecta. Its Web site is an ideal starting place to begin a search for information. The search process is easier because a wealth of information can be found in one place. Individuals with osteogenesis imperfecta and their families can get some basic information if they are unfamiliar with the condition or have been newly diagnosed. Teens and adults with osteogenesis imperfecta can get up-to-date information on genetic research, surgical options, and medications. It is a one-stop shop for people with osteogenesis imperfecta and their families. Included at the Web site are:

- Information about osteogenesis imperfecta
- Information about living with osteogenesis imperfecta
- Support groups
- Information about medical treatments
- Access to information fact sheets and a glossary of medical terms
- A News and Events page
- A chat room
- Links
- A Tell-a-Friend page
- The Foundation Store for items such as videos and books
- Information for medical and research professionals

The Osteogenesis Imperfecta Foundation's Web page also provides visitors with the opportunity to ask specific questions. This makes it easy to get the information you need in an easy to maneuver environment. Once you have the information you need or an idea of what you are looking for, you can search the Osteogenesis Imperfecta Foundation site or connect with some of the other links available on the site. In addition to the Web site information, the Foundation has numerous publications, books, and reprints of interest. Calling 800-981-2663 will put you in touch with people who have the answers you are looking for or who are able to put you in touch with someone who does.

Discussing the information you find with family members, doctors, or therapists can be valuable. Your healthcare team is one of the best sounding boards you have. Often the team members are aware of the latest information or have read about the current fads and can be very helpful in sorting out information that is often confusing or complex. Family members can provide valuable information about what may fit your family's life style. For those who are hesitant or feel that talking about such things with healthcare providers is out of the question, perhaps it's time to consider a new healthcare team.

Organizations that may have additional useful information on osteogenesis imperfecta are listed below with a short description, phone number, and Web address.

The **Osteogenesis Imperfecta Federation of Europe** (OIFE) aims to represent the interests of its European members. This site collects, publishes, and exchanges information on osteogenesis imperfecta. The OIFE tries to describe the problems of people with osteogenesis imperfecta to national or supranational organizations with the goal of improving accessibility and public health services. This organization also promotes research, surveys, and investigations on the causes, treatments, and effects of osteogenesis imperfecta. This web site provides information in several languages and links to the web sites of all member groups. www.oife.org

The **National Institutes of Health** (NIH) is the nation's federally funded premier organization for the study of disease and prevention. Its mission is science in pursuit of fundamental knowledge about the nature and behavior of living systems and the application of that knowledge to extend healthy life and reduce the burdens of illness and disability. The NIH has an osteogenesis imperfecta research program, and may provide information on the latest research on osteogenesis imperfecta. 301-496-4000. www.nih.gov

The **Alliance for Technology Access** (ATA) is a national organization dedicated to helping children and adults who have disabilities gain access to the benefits of adaptive technology. It has a nationwide network of community-based assistive technology resource centers, which may provide technology information for individuals with osteogenesis imperfecta. The national office can be reached by phone or via the Internet.707-778-3011. www.ataccess.org

The **American Academy of Orthopaedic Surgeons** (AAOS) provides educational and practice management services for orthopaedic surgeons and allied health professionals. The AAOS also serves as an advocate for improved patient care and informs the public about the science of orthopaedics. The patient education section of this Web site explains many surgical procedures and offers advice on bone health. It may provide resources for those in need of an orthopedist specializing in osteogenesis imperfecta in your community. 800-346-2267. www.aaos.org

The **American Academy of Pediatrics** (APA) is the professional association for pediatricians. On its Web site there are sections that provide information on a wide array of topics including Children's Health, Immunization, Car Safety Seats, and Books on Parenting. 847-434-4000. www.aap.org

The **American Dental Association** (ADA) is the professional association of dentists committed to the public's oral health, ethics, science, and professional advancement. The ADA focuses on advocacy, education, research, and the development of standards. The ADA may have information on dental research along with information on dental care for people with osteogenesis imperfecta. 312-440-2500. www.ada.org

The **American Medical Association** (AMA), a national association of physicians, has a Web page and a well respected medical journal, the *Journal of the American Medical Association* (*JAMA*). Both contain information of interest on many medical topics and concerns. 800-621-8335. www.ama-assn.org

The **American Occupational Therapy Association** (AOTA) advances the quality, availability, use, and support of occupational therapy through standard setting, advocacy, education, and research on behalf of its members and the public. Occupational therapy is a health and rehabilitation profession that helps people regain, develop, and build skills that are important for independent functioning, health, well-being, security, and happiness. It may provide resources for those in need of an occupational therapist specializing in osteogenesis imperfecta in your community. 301-652-2682. www.aota.org

The **American Physical Therapy Association** (APTA) is a national professional organization representing more than 63,000 members. Its mission, as the principal membership organization representing and promoting the profession of physical therapy, is to further the profession's role in the prevention, diagnosis, and treatment of movement dysfunctions and the enhancement of the physical health and functional abilities of members of the public. It may provide resources for those in need of a physical therapist specializing in osteogenesis imperfecta in your community. 800-999-2782. www.apta.org

The **American Society for Bone and Mineral Research** (ASBMR) is a professional, scientific, and medical society established to bring together clinical and experimental scientists involved in the study of bone and mineral metabolism. It encourages and promotes the study of this expanding field through annual scientific meetings, an official journal, the *Journal of Bone and Mineral Research,* advocacy, and interaction with government agencies and related societies. This web site includes an interactive section on bone biology that includes osteogenesis imperfecta. 202-367-1161. www.asbmr.org

Easter Seals provides a wide range of services to children and adults. Children's services help kids with disabilities succeed in school. Easter Seals employment programs help people learn job skills and enter the workplace. Easter Seals physical medicine and rehabilitation services help people return to their everyday lives. The services are comprehensive and individualized to meet each client's needs, family-focused to meet each family member's concerns, outcome-oriented with a goal of enhanced independence, and cost-effective through benefiting from public support. Resources for those in need of therapeutic services in a given area may be provided through a nationwide network of more than 450 service sites. This Web site provides information about national and local community programs. Many Easter Seals offices provide loaner car seats for infants and children in spica casts. 800-221-6827. www.easterseals.com

Genetic Information and Patient Services. This Web site offers a critical comparative study of Internet information concerning genetic disorders and birth defects. The frequently updated information is provided as a free public service by Genetic Information and Patient Services, Inc. 480-539-6063. www.icomm.ca/geneinfo

The **International Bone and Mineral Society** (IBMS) is a world-leading, scientific, nonprofit organization and a major international society for promoting the generation and dissemination of knowledge of basic biology and clinical science of the skeleton and mineral metabolism. It has more than 2,500 members representing 60 countries worldwide. In addition, the IBMS works closely with over 30 national and regional bone groups, expanding the IBMS network to over 10,000 professionals in the field. IBMS also engages in outreach to other medical specialties to increase interdisciplinary awareness and education. 202-367-1121. www.ibmsonline.org

Little People of America (LPA). This nonprofit organization provides support and information to people of short stature and their families. Here you'll find resources pertaining to dwarfism and LPA programs, medical data, instructions on how to join an e-mail discussion group, and links to numerous other dwarfism-related sites. 888-472-2001. www.lpaonline.org

March of Dimes. The mission of the March of Dimes is to improve the health of babies by preventing birth defects and infant mortality. Through their toll-free number, pregnancy information experts are ready to answer questions big and small. The March of Dimes advocates for health insurance for babies, children, and women. It may provide resources for those in need of perinatal health and insurance information. 888-663-4637. www.modimes.org

The **National Association of Children's Hospitals and Related Institutions** (NACHRI) is an organization of more than 160 hospitals that promotes the health and well-being of all children and their families through support of children's hospitals and health systems that are committed to excellence in providing healthcare to children. 703-684-1355. www.childrenshospitals.net

National Center on Physical Activity and Disability (NCPAD). Funded by the Centers for Disease Control and Prevention (www.cdc.gov), the NCPAD believes that exercise is for everyone. Having a disabling condition does not mean that one cannot be healthy. The NCPAD's mission is to encourage and support people with disabling conditions who wish to increase their overall level of activity and participate in any and all types of physical activity. The NCPAD offers a wide variety of resources to help people with disabling conditions become more active, including searchable databases, documents, and discussion groups, all providing up-to-date information. It may provide resources related to physical activity for people with osteogenesis imperfecta. 800-900-8086. www.ncpad.org

The **National Organization for Rare Disorders** (NORD) is a federation of voluntary health organizations, including the Osteogenesis Imperfecta Foundation. It is dedicated to improving the identification, treatment, and cure of rare disorders. It promotes education, research and advocacy. 203-744-0100. www.rarediseases.org.

The **National Osteoporosis Foundation** (NOF) is the leading nonprofit, voluntary health organization dedicated to promoting lifelong bone health in order to reduce the widespread prevalence of osteoporosis and associated fractures, while working to find a cure for the disease through programs of research, education, and advocacy. Adults with osteogenesis imperfecta may find this site particularly helpful. 202-223-2226. www.nof.org

Shriners Hospitals for Children is a network of 22 pediatric specialty hospitals where children under the age of 18 receive medical care free of charge. All of the orthopedic hospitals are equipped and staffed to treat children with congenital orthopedic deformities, problems resulting from orthopedic injuries, and diseases of the musculoskeletal system. Shriners Hospitals for Children may provide resources for those in need of orthopedic care for children with osteogenesis imperfecta near your community. The interdisciplinary team from the Shriners Hospital in Montreal has written a book about their experiences caring for children with osteogenesis imperfecta. *Interdisciplinary Treatment Approach for Children with Osteogenesis Imperfecta* is available for purchase through the Web site. The Shriners Hospitals in Chicago, Montreal, and many other cities have specific clinics devoted to the care of children with osteogenesis imperfecta. 800-237-5055 in the United States or 800-361-7256 in Canada. www.shrinershq.org

Many children's hospitals have Web sites that offer information about childhood illnesses as well as information about rare disorders such as osteogenesis imperfecta. Here are three examples:

Children's Hospital of Philadelphia (CHOP). This hospital web site offers a section titled "Your Child's Health," that is often mentioned in health education programs. It presents information on many topics that are important to parents. These include a Health and Wellness Center, an Index of Medical Conditions, and health tips on a variety of infant and child care topics. 215-590-3000. www.chop.edu

Texas Scottish Rite Hospital for Children (TSRHC). Expertise in the treatment of orthopedic conditions, certain related neurological disorders, and learning differences has gained the hospital national and international recognition. To find out the criteria needed to become a TSRHC patient, call the hospital. Resources for those in need of orthopedic care for children with osteogenesis imperfecta may be provided. 214-559-7477 or 800-421-1121, ext. 7477. www.tsrhc.org

The Bones Page. This Web site is administered by Horacio Plotkin, MD, Assistant Professor of Pediatrics and Orthopedic Surgery at the University of Nebraska College of Medicine and Medical Director of the Metabolic Bone Diseases Clinic at the University of Nebraska Medical Center and Children's Hospital in Omaha. It features tips for enhancing everyday life for children and adults with osteogenesis imperfecta and their families. www.geocities .com/CapeCanaveral/Lab/3608

Local services that may be available in your community include, but are not limited to, the following organizations: the Department of Public Health; the Department of Public Aid; the Department of Rehabilitation Services; and the Department of Vocational Rehabilitation Services, Division of Services for Children with Special Needs.

3. Support Services

Support can come from many different areas. At times a person may be able to provide support to others while at other times that person may need to receive it. Support comes from individuals, groups and organizations. Chat rooms, and list serves are increasingly popular Internet venues for support.

An underlying note of caution needs to permeate all of these areas: one size does not fit all. When contributing to a support group, what can you do to help? Be honest, be concise, and be available for follow-up questions. Follow the Health on the Net code. Do you have some information that you feel is important enough to share? Get signed up with the Osteogenesis Imperfecta Foundation chat room (www.oif.org), so that you can share it. Contact your local support group, hospital, and church or community group. Can you contribute to the pool of knowledge? You bet! Think of something that was shared with you and your family that made a difference in your life. Don't underestimate the importance of sharing even one small thing.

The Osteogenesis Imperfecta Foundation (800-981-2663; bonelink@ oif.org) has support groups across the country that are run by volunteers. When asked how they benefit from a group, members say they are looking for information on osteogenesis imperfecta, that they derive a sense of comfort through hearing from others who have had similar experiences, and it is a place where they can go to seek advice. Older people with osteogenesis imperfecta believe they can share their experiences with younger people, thus helping them to cope. And, at all levels, there is the desire for friendship and understanding. If you are interested in joining a support group, contact the Osteogenesis Imperfecta Foundation. Other types of support activities include the following:

One-on-One Support. The Foundation has staff and local volunteers who can provide support and information by telephone or e-mail. Contact the Foundation to request assistance and the name of a support volunteer whom you can call.

OI Foundation Key Pals Program. Young people aged 9 to 17 years who have osteogenesis imperfecta and are interested in having a pen pal are invited to join the Osteogenesis Imperfecta Foundation's Key Pals Program. Although most participants correspond by e-mail, "snail mail" users can also be accommodated. To request an application, contact the Foundation.

Some other groups that offer support include:

Family Voices. This national grassroots network of families and friends, advocates for healthcare services that are family-centered, community-based, comprehensive, and coordinated for all children and youth with special healthcare needs. It promotes the inclusion of all families as decision makers at all levels of healthcare; and supports essential partnerships between families and professionals. One of Family Voices' key missions is to help families locate all programs within their state that could provide assistance, including financial assistance to children with chronic health issues. 888-835-5669. www.familyvoices.org

The Genetic Alliance, formerly called the Alliance of Genetic Support Groups, is an international coalition consisting of millions of people with genetic conditions and more than 600 advocacy, research, and healthcare organizations that represent their interests. As a broad-based coalition of key stakeholders, the Alliance builds partnerships to promote healthy lives for those living with genetic conditions. With a 16-year history as a 501(c)(3) not-for-profit organization, the Alliance identifies solutions to emerging problems and endeavors to reduce obstacles to rapid and effective translation of research into accessible technologies and services. The Osteogenesis Imperfecta Foundation is a member of the Genetic Alliance. 202-966-5557. www.geneticalliance.org

For additional support services information, please see Appendixes C and D.

4. Educational Materials

Where else can you look for information? There is an abundance of information within the healthcare environment. The range of resources runs from newspapers and magazines to Web sites and medical journals. The source of all medical information as well as the audience it was prepared for needs to be considered. Using the National Library of Medicine Web site (www.nlm.nih.gov) you can enter PubMed to track down what has been published about osteogenesis imperfecta in reputable print and on-line medical journals such as the *Journal of the American Medical Association (JAMA),* the *New England Journal of Medicine (N Engl J Med)* or the *Journal of Bone and Joint Surgery (J Bone Joint Surg).* A summary or abstract is provided and in some cases a link to the journal's Web site. Occasionally, the complete article will be available free of charge, but more often a subscription to the print journal or the on-line service is required. Some journals allow the Internet customer to purchase individual articles. Policies vary greatly, but subscriptions and single article prices can be quite expensive.

Libraries are excellent sources of free or low-cost information. Public libraries often have a research librarian on staff who is available to help customers learn how to access the system. Some large library systems have a branch library designated as a health information center. Some universities, medical schools or medical centers are open to members of the public too. The local public library is a good place to begin. Think of the library as a one-stop shop. Most public libraries have print media, newspapers, magazines, journals, pamphlets, textbooks, video/audio tapes, CD-ROMs, and the Internet. Most libraries are able to get reprints of journal or other articles for a small fee. There are also interlibrary loan services, which allow you to review recent journals and books for a short time, typically for a small fee.

When considering the merit of material in medical and scientific journals, as well as in other publications that draw on them, such as brochures and newsletters, it is important to know what type of journal it is. In general, there are two types, peer reviewed or non-peer reviewed. Peer reviewed journals tend to have articles that undergo scientific scrutiny by experts in their respective fields. The articles may be written in scientific terms for medical and scientific professionals and may be hard to read for everyone. Additionally, the information reported in journal articles may refer to experimental procedures that are not yet available to patients outside of the study or approved for human studies. Non-peer reviewed publications include magazines, newspapers, and newsletters whose intended audience is the general public. It may be useful to discuss the information reported in studies with the physician responsible for the care of the person with osteogenesis imperfecta.

Reviewing research, information, and scientific studies specific to osteogenesis imperfecta is a good starting point. Utilizing reliable sources of information and institutions is invaluable. Additionally, libraries are a good back-up when your home computer crashes or you need an emergency source for Web surfing or to get your e-mail.

Web sites can also be sources of medical information. As mentioned above, the National Library of Medicine MedlinePlus site is very comprehensive. Another popular site is WebMD.

WebMD. The mission of this site's organizers is to bring you the most objective, trustworthy, and accurate health information on the Web. Their daily goal is to ensure that WebMD is a practical and relevant content source for health and medicine. They are committed to providing information on a wide variety of health topics. Rather than filtering certain types of information that may or may not apply to an individual's personal health, they rely on the reader to choose the information that is most appropriate. 201-703-3400. www.webmd.com

Books are another good source of information, not only about osteogenesis impefecta itself, but also about the many issues related to living with osteogenesis imperfecta and raising a child with special needs. Publications from Woodbine Press include books on various disability issues for young children and parents. The magazine *Exceptional Parent* both in print and on its Web site includes reviews of books for children and adults on many relevant topics.

Several books are currently available through the Osteogenesis Imperfecta Foundation and additional titles are added each year:
* *Growing Up With OI–A Guide for Children*
* *Growing Up With OI–A Guide for Families and Caregivers*
* *Therapeutic Strategies for Osteogenesis Imperfecta: A Guide for Physical Therapists and Occupational Therapists*
* *Managing OI: A Medical Manual*
* *OI: A Guide for Nurses*
* *Jason's First Day!*

For additional information please see Appendixes A, E, and F.

5. Resources for Devices and Adaptive Equipment

Thousands of sources from which to obtain medical and adaptive equipment exist; catalogues, Web sites, television, magazines, and word of mouth are just a few. Important points to consider when looking into adaptive equipment for your child or yourself include:

• Each child has unique needs; one size does not necessarily fit every child.

• Keep an open mind.

• Try it before you buy it whenever possible. Items such as braces, wheelchairs, and splints must fit perfectly. Just as you do when you buy new clothing, you need to try it on to see if it fits. In the case of a new piece of power equipment, just as in buying a new car, take it for a test drive before you make the purchase.

• Whenever possible, include the physician and physical or occupational therapist in your assessment and decision making process to order complex equipment. Just as important, have them check equipment with you and your child at the time and place that the vendor delivers it.

• Be creative. After a need has been identified, it is often possible for the parent and therapist to modify an existing piece of equipment such as beds, tables, chairs, or toilets to suit the child with osteogenesis imperfecta. Everything does not necessarily need to come from a medical supply company.

As a parent, keeping yourself updated on the latest information about new equipment and adaptations can greatly improve a child's quality of life and your peace of mind. Healthcare providers, especially physical and occupational therapists should be the first line of information about adaptive equipment. Other resources include the Osteogenesis Imperfecta Foundation, special recreation associations, Easter Seals, Shriners Hospitals for Children, Special Olympics, resource guides from publications like *Exceptional Parent* magazine, and parents of children with osteogenesis imperfecta. Additional places to look for equipment information include the Internet, special needs magazines, local rehabilitation and therapy departments in hospitals and clinics, school districts, park districts, medical supply and product catalogues, and equipment vendors. Which product is right for your child depends on fit, affordability, versatility, and personal choice. Additional information regarding adaptive equipment resources is available in Appendixes B, E, H, and I.

6. Funding Resources

Funding for children with special needs is often available. Many funding sources are often overlooked and most are poorly advertised. A number of general funding sources may require investment of a bit of time to find and use, while others just require good old-fashioned asking for help.

A number of national and local organizations have resources for children with special needs; a selection is listed below. Other sources of funding information include your pediatrician, occupational and physical therapists, the social service department at your children's hospital or the hospital your child uses, and the public health department. In some cases, the Osteogenesis Imperfecta Foundation can put you in touch with organizations and others who can provide sources of funding for you and your child. In addition, word of mouth and personal contacts made by friends and therapists are also a good place to start.

Family Voices is a grass roots organization that is committed to helping families locate and understand all areas of support available in their states for children with chronic health challenges. Its Web site (www.familyvoices.org) links to its network of state representatives and includes lists of up-to-date contacts for state agencies and programs. Information is also provided about helping young people make the transition to adult services.

Individuals with Disabilities Education Act (IDEA). The IDEA requires all states and territories to provide early intervention and preschool education for children with disabilities and special healthcare needs. The infant and toddler programs that serve children from birth to age three are referred to as Part C programs, and the preschool special education programs that serve children from age three to five are known as 619 programs. Information on state-specific programs can be obtained at the National Early Childhood Technical Assistance Center (NECTAC) Web site, www.nectas.unc.edu. Parent Training and Information (PTI) centers also provide information on this and other education-related topics. Call 800-695-0285 or visit www.taalliance.org/centers for information about the PTI program in each community.

Infinitec. The mission of Infinitec is to advance independence and promote inclusive opportunities for children and adults with disabilities through technology. The Infinitec staff helps people with disabilities find and get access to information, technology services, training, assistive equipment, and specialists by creating partnerships that maximize resources. 312-368-0308. www.infinitec.org

Technical Assistance Alliance Coordinating Office. Training centers in each state provide training and information for parents of infants, toddlers, school-aged children, and young adults with disabilities as well as the professionals who work with their families. The Alliance Coordinating Office provides information on these programs and can be reached at 888-248-0822 or www.taalliance.org.

Title V Programs. These are available in each state and are funded, in part, through the federal Title V Block Grant that provides health-related services to children with special healthcare needs and their families. Financial eligibility, residency criteria, and medical eligibility criteria vary from state to state, as does the name of the program. Information can be obtained from the Institute for Child Health Policy Web site, www.ichp.edu.

Variety–The Children's Charity. Its mission is to provide life-saving and life-enriching assistance to children challenged by physical and mental disabilities, poverty, abuse, and neglect through grants, scholarships, cultural enrichment programs, outreach activities and other donations. Variety will sometimes pay for specific pieces of adaptive equipment in certain regions of the United States. 888-852-1300. www.usvariety.org

Local church organizations are also places to consider for some financial support through bake sales, car washes, and other fundraisers.

Individual state organizations, including the Department of Rehabilitation Services, the Department of Vocational Rehabilitation, and the Department of Public Aid, may also provide support. In general the services are available to working individuals from 16 to 64 years of age. Vocational rehabilitation can often assist with driver training, car or van modifications, and tuition assistance. Individual states may have specific eligibility criteria or require a certain level of income and level of need or disability. A letter of medical necessity from your physician and physical or occupational therapist for services or equipment provided may also be required. It is a good idea to check with your state organization to determine its specific eligibility criteria.

The **Americans with Disabilities Act** (ADA) gives civil rights protection to persons with disabilities similar to those provided on the basis of race, color, sex, national origin, age, and religion. It guarantees equal opportunity for persons with disabilities in public accommodations, employment, transportation, state and local government services, and telecommunications. www.usdoj.gov/crt/ada.

Many states have technical and assistive technology resource Web sites. These sites can be accessed by plugging the terms "technical assistance" or "assistive technology" into a search engine such as Google. One such Web site is the Michigan Assistive Technology Resource.

Michigan Assistive Technology Resource (MATR). The overall purpose of the MATR is to provide information services, support materials, technical assistance, and training to local and intermediate school districts in Michigan to increase their capacity to address the needs of students with disabilities for assistive technology. MATR Services Information provides details about state-of-the-art technology, daily living devices, equipment, and the identification of assistive technology solutions for children with disabilities. Information requests are received by MATR staff via telephone, electronic mail, fax, and US mail. The staff researches resources and provides current information on products, services, and service providers in the field of assistive technology. MATR also maintains a collection of catalogues, reprints, and publications to help assistive technology personnel in the schools. 800-274-7426. www.cenmi.org/matr/aboutus.asp.

Additional funding sources are listed in Appendix D.

7. Sports and Recreation

Many sources of information relating to sports and recreation are discussed in Chapter 6. Additional sports and recreation resources, including information on therapeutic recreation, child life, and the Blaze Sports Clubs of America, are listed below in Appendix F.

8. Appendixes

Appendix A. *Information Credibility*

One Web site that has taken information credibility seriously is **MedlinePlus** (www.medlineplus.gov), which has very specific selection criteria for what goes onto the site. MedlinePlus helps consumers find health information by providing access to a number of authoritative databases, including the National Library of Medicine, the National Institutes of Health, Medline (a database that indexes medical literature), and ClinicalTrials.gov.

The selection guidelines used by MedlinePlus to evaluate links to Web pages are listed below.

• Quality, authority, and accuracy of content. The source of the content is established, respected, and dependable. A list of advisory board members or consultants is published on the site. The content is appropriate to the audience level, well organized, and easy to use. The information is from primary resources (for example, textual material, abstracts, and Web pages). Lists of links are evaluated and reviewed and quality-filtered.

• The purpose of the Web page is educational and is not selling a product or service. Most content is available at no charge.

• Availability and maintenance of the Web page. The Web site is consistently available. Links from the site are maintained. The source for the contents of the Web page(s) and the entity responsible for maintaining the Web site (Webmaster, organization, and creator of the content) are clear. Information is current or an update date is included. Registration is not required to view the information on the site.

• Special features. The site provides unique information on the topic with a minimum of redundancy and overlap between resources. The site contains special features such as graphics/diagrams, glossary, or other unique information. The content of the site is accessible to persons with disabilities.

Hi-Ethics (www.hiethics.com) is another company that has taken the next step forward in the health information arena. Also known as Health Internet Ethics, it was formed to address privacy, advertising and content quality issues for Internet health consumers. Member companies readily donated the skills and knowledge of their executive leadership to develop their own set of principles. Hi-Ethics companies provide on-line health services that reflect

high quality and ethical standards with the following goals:
- Providing health information that is trustworthy and up to date
- Clearly identifying on-line advertising and disclosing sponsorships or other financial relationships that significantly affect our content or services
- Keeping personal information private and secure, and employing special precautions for any personal health information
- Empowering consumers to distinguish on-line health services that follow Hi-Ethics principles from those that do not

As Hi-Ethics reports, "the Internet provides unprecedented potential for enhancing the quality of and access to healthcare information and resources. The Internet offers a wealth of information that can help patients learn about their medical conditions and engage in more productive discussions with their healthcare providers. It also offers convenience unmatched in the off-line world. At the same time, the enormous potential of the Internet for healthcare brings with it enormous risks, such as inaccurate or biased articles or the abuse of personal information. The companies came together to develop the Hi-Ethics principles because consumers need to distinguish trustworthy health Web sites from others."

Another credible information source is **PubMed**. A service of the National Library of Medicine, it includes over 14 million citations for biomedical articles back to the 1950s. PubMed includes links to many sites providing full text articles and other related resources. www.ncbi.nih.gov/entrez/query.fcgi.

The **Cochrane Collaboration** (www.cochrane.org) is an international nonprofit and independent organization, dedicated to making up-to-date, accurate information about the effects of healthcare readily available worldwide. It produces and disseminates systematic reviews of healthcare interventions and promotes the search for evidence in the form of clinical trials and other studies of interventions.

Appendix B. *Devices and Adaptive Equipment*

Please note that this list is intended to provide examples of a wide range of products that might be useful for a person who has osteogenesis imperfecta and his or her therapist. It is not an exhaustive list because of the sheer number of products available.

Splinting and bracing

Ace Bandages	888-232-2737 www.bd.com/elastics
AliMed Medical Supplies	800-225-2610 www.alimed.com
Benik Vests/Supports	800-442-8910 www.benik.com
North Coast	800-821-9319 www.northcoastmedical.com
Sammons Preston Rolyan	800-323-5547 www.sammonspreston.com
Southpaw Medical Supply	800-228-1698 www.southpawenterprises.com

Standing

EasyStand	800-342-8968 www.easystand.com
Granstand	800-827-8263 www.primeengineering.com
Mulholland	805-525-7165 www.mulhollandinc.com
Rifton Equipment	800-777-4244 www.rifton.com
Snug Seat	800-336-7684 www.snugseat.com
TherAdapt	800-261-4919 www.theradapt.com
Tumble Forms/Sammons Preston	800-323-5547 www.sammonspreston.com

Seating, positioning, and hygiene

Adaptive Mall for Children with Special Needs	800-371-2778 www.adaptivemall.com
Boppy	888-772-6779 www.boppy.com
Invacare	800-333-6900 www.invacare.com
Kaye Products	919-732-6444 www.Kayeproducts.com
Mulholland	805-525-7165 www.mulhollandinc.com
Peg Perego	800-671-1701 www.perego.com
Rifton Equipment	800-777-4244 www.rifton.com
ROHO/Crown Therapeutics	800-851-3449 www.therohogroup.com
Snug Seat	800-336-7684 www.snugseat.com
Sunrise Medical	888-333-2572 www.sunrisemedical.com
TherAdapt	800-261-4919 www.theradapt.com
Tumble Forms/Sammons Preston	800-323-5547 www.sammonspreston.com

Strollers

Convaid	800-552-1020 www.convaid.com
Maclaren	877-442-4622 www.maclarenbaby.com
Mulholland	805-525-7165 www.mulhollandinc.com
Ortho Kinetics	800-558-7786 www.ez-international.com
Otto Bock	800-328-4058 www.ottobockus.com

Peg Perego	800- 671-1701
	www.perego.com
Quickie Kid Cart	888-333-2572
	www.sunrisemedical.com
Snug Seat	800-336-7684
	www.snugseat.com
Tumble Forms/Sammons Preston	800-323-5547
	www.sammonspreston.com

Power wheelchairs and scooters

Amigo Mobility Scooters	800-692-6446
	www.myamigo.com
Bruno	800-882-8768
	www.bruno.com
Freedom Designs	800-331-8551
	www.freedomdesigns.com
Invacare	800-333-6900
	www.invacare.com
Levo	888-538-6872
	www.levousa.com
Motion Concepts	888-433-6818
	www.motionconcepts.com
Natural Access Beach Wheelchairs	800-411-7789
	www.landeez.com
Permobil	800-736-0925
	www.permobilusa.com
Pride	800-800-8586
	www.pridemobility.com
Quickie	888-333-2572
	www.sunrisemedical.com
Snug Seat	800-336-7684
	www.snugseat.com
WheelchairNet	412-383-6793
	www.wheelchairnet.org

Power mobility conversion

Frank Mobility Systems: Emotion/Efix	888-426-8581
	www.frankmobility.com
Johnson & Johnson/Independence Technology I-Glide	877-794-4583
	www.ibotnow.com
Quickie	888-333-2572
	www.sunrisemedical.com

Bikes

Ambucs/Amtryke Specialty Bikes	336-869-2166
	www.ambucs.com/aamtryke.htm
Creative Mobility Bikes	800-711-2453
	www.creativemobility.net
CycleTote Bike Trailer	800-747-2407
	www.cycletote.com
Freedom Concept Bikes	800-661-9915
	www.freedomconcepts.com
Infinitec	312-368-0380
	www.infinitec.org
Lightning Hand Cycles	805-736-0700
	www.lightningbikes.com
Moto Med/Great Lakes Medical	708-386-6501
	www.greatlakesmedical.com
Power Trainer Hand/Leg Cycle	800-852-6869
	www.scifit.com
Saratoga Hand Cycle	800-474-4010
	www.randscot.com
Step'n Go Cycle	800-648-7335
	www.stepngo.com

Mobile standers

Davis Made/Standing Dani	810-742-0581
	www.standingdani.com
EasyStand Standers	800-342-8968
	www.easystand.com
Kaye Products	919-732-6444
	www.Kayeproducts.com

Lite Gait	800-332-9255
	www.litegait.com
Mulholland	805-525-7165
	www.mulhollandinc.com
Rifton Equipment	800-777-4244
	www.rifton.com
Snug Seat	800-336-7684
	www.snugseat.com

Manual scooters

Creepster Crawler	800-577-1317
	www.redbarn-enter.com
Fisher-Price	800-432-5437
	www.fisher-price.com/us
Radio Flyer Wagons	800-621-7613
	www.radioflyer.com
Star Car	800-463-5685
	www.tashinc.com
Step 2 Children's Toys	800-347-8372
	www.step2.com

Car seats

BESI Restraining Harness	800-543-8222
	www.besi-inc.com
Britax	888-427-4829
	www.britaxusa.com
Carrie Car Seat	800-371-2778
	www.tumbleforms.com
Columbia Car Seat	800-454-6612
	www.columbiamedical.com
Dream Ride Car Seat/Car Bed	800-544-1108
	www.coscojuvenile.com
EZ-On Vest	800-323-6598
	www.ezonpro.com
Graco	800-345-4109
	www.gracobaby.com

Kid-EZB Transit Model/Sunrise	888-333-2572 www.sunrisemedical.com
Mulholland Growth Guidance	805-525-7165 www.mulhollandinc.com
Peg Perego	800-671-1701 www.perego.com
Snug Seat/Britax	800-336-7684 www.snugseat.com

Car or van modifications

Braun	800-843-5438 www.braunlift.com
Bruno	800-882-8768 www.bruno.com
Creative Mobility Vans	619-474-4072 www.creativemobility.com
Daimler/Chrysler Automobility Program	800-255-9877 www.dc-automobility.com
Ford Motor Company	800-952-2248 www.mobilitymotoringprogram.com
Freedom Driving Aids	888-605-9999 www.freedomdrivingaids.com
General Motors	800-323-9935 www.GMmobility.com
Independent Mobility Systems	800-467-8267 www.Rampvan.net
Volkswagen	800-374-8389 www.VW.com

Bathing and hygiene

Aquatec/Dolomite	888-347-4537 www.clarkehealthcare.com
Arjo	800-323-1245 www.arjo.com
Columbia Bath Equipment	800-454-6612 www.columbiamedical.com

Guardian   800-333-4000
                                            www.sunrisemedical.com
Rifton Equipment   800-777-4244
                                            www.rifton.com

Transfer and lift devices

Arjo   800-323-1245
                                            www.arjo.com
Barrier Free Lifts   800-582-8732
                                            www.barrierfreelifts.com
Horcher Lifting Systems   800-582-8732
                                            www.horcher.com
Hoyer/Guardian   800-333-4000
                                            www.sunrisemedical.com
Medi-Man   800-868-0441
                                            www.bhm-medical.com
Multi-Lift/Access Unlimited   800-849-2143
                                            www.accessunlimited.com
SureHands Lifts   800-724-5305
                                            www.surehands.com

Beds and cribs

Hard Manufacturing   800-873-4273
                                            www.hardmfg.com
Hertz Supply/Volker Beds   800-321-4240
                                            www.hertzsupply.com
Invacare   800-333-6900
                                            www.invacare.com

Clothing

Finally It Fits   866-866-9740
                                            www.finallyitfits.com

Aquatics

My Pool Pal Flotation Swimwear   800-715-9435
                                            www.mypoolpal.com

Sprint Aquatic Products	800-235-2156
	www.sprintaquatics.com

Working pets

Canine Companions	800-572-2275
	www.caninecompanions.org
Paws With a Cause	800-253-7297
	www.pawswithacause.org

Adaptive toys

Play With a Purpose	888-330-1826
	www.playwithapurpose.com
Sammons Preston Rolyan	800-323-5547
	www.sammonspreston.com

Wheelchair stair climbing and stair glides

Bruno	800-882-8768
	www.bruno.com
Frank Mobility Systems	888-426-8581
	www.frankmobility.com
Garaventa	800-663-6556
	www.garaventa.ca
Johnson & Johnson/Independence Technology I-Glide	877-794-4583
	www.ibotnow.com

Augmentative communication

Alpha Smart	888-274-0680
	www2.alphasmart.com
Dynavox/Sunrise Medical	800-333-4000
	www.sunrisemedical.com
Prentke Romich Company	800-262-1984
	www.prentrom.com
Tuff Talker/Freedom Toughbook	800-869-8521
	www.words-plus.com

Assistive devices and gait trainers

Davis Made/Standing Dani	810-742-0581
	www.standingdani.com
Guardian	800-333-4000
	www.sunrisemedical.com
Kaye Products	919-732-6444
	www.kayeproducts.com
Mulholland	805-525-7165
	www.mulhollandinc.com
Rifton Equipment	800-777-4244
	www.rifton.com
Snug Seat	800-336-7684
	www.snugseat.com
Walk Easy	800-441-2904
	www.walkeasy.com
Wenzelite	800-706-9255
	www.wenzelite.com

There is a "virtual" tour of products available through the **World Congress and Exposition on Disabilities** at www.wcdexpo.com. For more information about the World Congress go to the site or call 877-923-3976. The Abilities EXPO travels to several cities around the country throughout the year and has a number of equipment vendors showing their products and services. For information you can go to www.abilitiesexpo.com or call 800-385-3085. The **MedTrade** show is the largest trade show of medical, home health, and personal medical care products in the country. For information go to www.medtrade.com or call 800-933-8735.

Home modifications

Making modifications to one's home is also an area that can be important to a family with osteogenesis imperfecta. The following centers are good places to start looking for information:

The **Center for Universal Design**, at North Carolina State University, Raleigh, is a national research, information, and technical assistance center. Its staff develops and advocates for universal design in housing and in public and commercial buildings. 800-647-6777. www.design.ncsu.edu/cud

The **National Resource Center on Supportive Housing and Home Modifications** is based at the University of Southern California, Los Angeles. It promotes home modifications that enhance the ability of people of all ages and abilities to live independently. 213-740-1364. www.homemods.org

Appendix C. Federally Funded National Organizations for People with Special Needs

Several federally funded national organizations provide information and resources for people with special needs, including the following:

- ABLEDATA, a database on assistive technology products and rehabilitation equipment maintained for the National Institute on Disability and Rehabilitation Research. 800-227-0216. www.abledata.com
- Education Resource Information Center (ERIC) Clearinghouse on Disabilities and Gifted Children. 800-538-3742. www.eric.ed.gov
- National Association for the Education of Young Children (NAEYC). 800-424-2460. www.naeyc.org
- National Clearinghouse on Postsecondary Education for Individuals with Disabilities. 800-554-3284. www.heath.gwu.edu
- National Health Information Center (NHIC). 800-336-4797. www.health.gov/nhic
- National Information Center for Children and Youth with Disabilities (NICHCY). 800-695-0285. www.nichcy.org
- National Rehabilitation Information Center (NARIC). 800-346-2742. www.naric.com
- Office of Special Education and Rehabilitative Services (OSERS). 202-245-7468. www.ed.gov/offices/OSERS

Appendix D. Funding and Advocacy Groups

Athletes Helping Athletes 888-566-5221
www.roadrunnersports.com

Children's Hopes and Dreams Foundation 973-361-7366
www.childrenswishes.org

Children's Wish Foundation International 800-323-9474
www.childrenswish.org

Disabled Children's Relief Fund 516-377-1605
www.dcrf.com

Elks Clubs of the United States 773-755-4700
www.elks.org

First Hand Foundation 816-201-1569
www.firsthandfoundation.org

Grant a Wish Children's Promise Foundation 800-933-5470
www.grant-a-wish.org

Grants and Related Resources 517-432-6123
www.lib.msu.edu/harris23/grants/servicec.htm

HEATH Resource Center of the American 800-544-3284
Council on Education www.heath.gwu.edu

Jaycees US Headquarters 800-529-2337
www.usjaycees.org

Kiwanis International 317-875-8755
www.kiwanis.org

Lions Clubs International 630-571-5466
www.lionsclubs.org

Make a Wish Foundation 800-722-9474
www.wish.org

National Association of Children's Hospitals and 703-684-1355
Related Institutions www.childrenshospitals.net

Ronald McDonald House Charities 630-623-7048
www.rmhc.com

Rotary International 847-866-3000
www.rotary.org

Starlight Foundation 310-479-1212
www.slsb.org

Sunshine Foundation	800-767-1976
	www.sunshinefoundation.org
The Dream Factory	800-456-7556
	www.dreamfactoryinc.com

College resources

The HEATH Resource Center of the American Council on Education is a national clearinghouse on postsecondary education for individuals with disabilities. Its publications are updated yearly and are available both in print and on-line (e-mail HEATH@ace.nche.edu). Of special interest are the publications *Financial Aid for Students with Disabilities* and *Vocational Rehabilitation Services: A Consumer Guide for Postsecondary Students.* 800-544-3284. www.heath.gwu.edu

Another excellent book and a great starting place for information on college funding is *The Scholarship Book 2000: The Complete Guide to Private-Sector Scholarships, Grants and Loans for Undergraduates* by Daniel J. Cassidy (Prentice Hall Press).

Advocacy groups

American Association of Persons with Disabilities	800-840-8844
	www.aapd-dc.org
Americans with Disabilities Act	800-514-0301
	www.usdoj.gov/crt/ada
Architectural and Transportation Barriers Compliance Board/US Access Board	800-872-2253
	www.access-board.gov
Association of University Centers on Disabilities	301-588-8252
	www.aucd.org
Children's Defense Fund	800-233-1200
	www.childrensdefense.org
Council for Exceptional Children	888-232-7733
	www.cec.sped.org
Disability Rights Education and Defense Fund	510-644-2555
	www.dredf.org
Family Voices	888-835-5669
	www.familyvoices.org

National Association of Protection and Advocacy Systems	202-408-9514 www.napas.org
National Family Caregivers Association	800-896-3650 www.nfcacares.org
Osteogenesis Imperfecta Foundation	800-981-2663 www.oif.org
Special Needs Advocate for Parents	888-310-9889 www.snapinfo.org

Appendix E. Magazines, Medical Journals, and Other Publications

The following magazines and reports have information specific to people with osteogenesis imperfecta and others with special needs:

Ability Magazine covers such topics as advocacy, parenting and family issues, assistive technology, employment, and nutrition and fitness.

949-854-8700
www.abilitymagazine.com

Abilities Magazine, a publication of the Canadian Abilities Foundation, contains reports and links for people with disabilities. 416-923-1885
www.enablelink.org or www.abilities.ca

Access to Travel provides information on travel, tours, and cruises for people with special needs. 303-232-2979
www.access-able.com

Active Living Magazine has articles on health, fitness, and recreation for people with disabilities. 905-957-6016
www.activelivingmagazine.com

Breakthrough, a newsletter published by the Osteogenesis Imperfecta Foundation, contains information specific to people with osteogenesis imperfecta and their families. 800-981-2663
www.oif.org

Careers and the disAbled is a career recruitment magazine published by Equal Opportunity Publications. www.eop.com

Challenge Magazine is published by Disabled Sports USA. www.dsusa.org

Hearing Health, a magazine with information on hearing loss, tinnitus, and assistive devices, is published by the Deafness Research Foundation.

800-829-5934
www.hearinghealthmag.com

Mainstream is a magazine with news about advocacy and life style issues.
www.mainstream-mag.com

New Mobility is a magazine with information on sports, travel, and recreation.
www.newmobility.com

Open World, a magazine with information on travel, is published by the Society for Accessible Travel and Hospitality.
212-447-7284
www.sath.org

Palaestra, a magazine listing resources on sports, physical education, and recreation for people who have a disability, is published by Challenge Publications.
309-833-1902
www.palaestra.com

Sports and Spokes, a magazine published by the Paralyzed Veterans of America, contains information on sports, recreation, equipment, and people.
888-888-2201
www.sns-magazine.com

Additionally, several special needs magazines publish yearly buyer's guides that provide a summary of goods and services available with contact information. These are good ready-reference books to keep in your personal library. The following magazines publish such guides:

Active Living Magazine
905-957-6016
www.activelivingmagazine.com

Biomechanics
415-947-6000
www.cmp.com

Exceptional Parent
877-372-7368
www.exceptionalparent.com

PT—Magazine of Physical Therapy
800-999-2782
www.apta.org

Rehab and Therapy Products Review
714-998-6242
www.rtproductsreview.com

The book *Assistive Technology for Persons with Disabilities,* by W. C. Mann and J. P. Lane (American Occupational Therapy Association, 1995) is a treasury of resources on technology, gadgets, and innovations.

Medical Journals

Medical journals that may have relevant information for people with osteogenesis imperfecta include the following:

American Journal of Physical Medicine and Rehabilitation	www.amjphysmedrehab.com
Journal of Bone and Joint Surgery	www.ejbjs.org
Journal of Pediatric Orthopaedics	www.pedorthopaedics.com
Journal of the American Medical Association	www.jama.ama-assn.org
Journal of the American Occupational Therapy Association	www.aota.org/ajot/index.asp
Journal of the American Physical Therapy Association	www.ptjournal.org
New England Journal of Medicine	www.nejm.org

Appendix F. Sports, Recreation, and Activity Camps

American Therapeutic Recreation Association	703-683-9420 www.atra-tr.org
Coalition of Child Life and Therapeutic Recreation Professionals	813-893-6265 www.childlife.org
National Recreation and Park Association	703-858-0784 www.nrpa.org
Paralympic Games	719-866-2030 www.usparalympics.org
Therapeutic Recreation	304-599-6465 www.recreationtherapy.com

Blaze Sports Clubs of America is a national community-based sports and fitness program for children and adults with disabilities that is a direct legacy of the 1996 Olympics held in Atlanta, Georgia.   770-850-8199
www.blazesports.com

Sports, Everyone! Recreation and Sports for the Physically Challenged of All Ages, published in 1995, is available from Conway Greene Publishing.   800-977-2665
www.conwaygreene.com

Activity camps

The American Camp Association (ACA) is a community of camp professionals dedicated to enriching the lives of children and adults through the camp experience. ACA members join together to share knowledge and experience and to ensure the quality of camp programs. The ACA publishes a guide to ACA-accredited camps with listings for specialized activities along with a listing of state contacts. Its Web site also has information on preparing for camp, articles for kids about camps, and information on choosing a camp for your child. Additionally there is a listing for special travel, tour, and adventure camps for people with special needs. 765-342-8456. www.acacamps.org. Also see Chapter 6.

Appendix G. Travel Information and Driving Programs

Access-Able Travel Agency	303-232-2979
	www.access-able.com
Access for Disabled Americans	925-284-6444
	www.accessfordisabled.com
Disability Travel and Recreation Resources	800-846-4537
	www.makoa.org/travel.htm
Emerging Horizons Accessible Travel News	209-599-9409
	www.emerginghorizons.com
National Center on Accessibility	812-856-4422
	www.indiana.edu/~nca/
Paralyzed Veterans of America	800-444-0120
	www.pva.org
Society for Accessible Travel and Hospitality	212-447-7284
	www.sath.org
Wheelchair Getaways	800-642-2042
	www.wheelchairgetaways.com

Driving programs

Association for Driver Rehabilitation Specialists	800-290-2344
	www.driver-ed.org
Infinite Potential Through Assistive Technology	312-368-0380
	www.infinitec.org

Appendix H. Quick Phone Number Reference List

Abilities Expo	800-385-3085
Abilities Magazine	416-923-1885
Ability Magazine	949-854-8700
ABLEDATA	800-227-0216
Access-Able Travel Agency	303-232-2979
Access for Disabled Americans	925-284-6444
Access to Travel Magazine	303-232-2979
Access Unlimited	800-849-2143
Ace Bandages	888-232-2737
Active Living Magazine	905-957-6016
Adaptive Mall for Children with Special Needs	800-371-2778
AliMed Medical Supplies	800-225-2610
Alliance for Technology Access	707-778-3011
Alpha Smart	888-274-0680
Ambucs/Amtryke Specialty Bikes	336-869-2166
American Academy of Orthopaedic Surgeons	800-346-2267
American Academy of Pediatrics	847-434-4000
American Association of Persons with Disabilities	800-840-8844
American Camp Association	765-342-8456
American Dental Association	312-440-2500
American Discount Medical Supplies	800-877-9100
American Medical Association	800-621-8335
American Occupational Therapy Association	301-652-2682
American Physical Therapy Association	800-999-2782
American Society for Bone and Mineral Research	202-367-1161
Americans with Disabilities Act Information	800-514-0301
American Therapeutic Recreation Association	703-683-9420
Amigo Mobility Scooters	800-692-6446
Aquatech/Dolomite Bath Lifts	800-347-4537
Architectural and Transportation Barriers Compliance Board/US Access Board	800-872-2253
Arjo Bath Lifts	800-323-1245
Association for Driver Rehabilitation Specialists	800-290-2344
Association of University Centers on Disabilities	301-588-8252

Athletes Helping Athletes	888-566-5221
Baby Abby	800-972-7357
Barrier Free Lifts	800-582-8732
Benick Vests/Supports	800-442-8910
BESI Restraining Harness	800-543-8222
Bike Rack Specialty Bikes	800-711-2453
Biomechanics Magazine	415-947-6000
Blaze Sports Clubs of America	770-850-8199
Boppy	888-772-6779
Braun	800-843-5438
***Breakthrough* (OI Foundation Newsletter)**	**800-981-2663**
Britax Car Seats	888-427-4829
Bruno	800-882-8768
Canine Companions	800-572-2275
Cardon Rehabilitation Products	800-944-7868
Care Medical Supply	800-443-7091
Carrie Car Seat	800-371-2778
Cascade DAFO Orthoses	800-848-7332
Center for Universal Design	800-647-6777
Centers for Disease Control	800-311-3435
Children's Defense Fund	800-233-1200
Children's Hopes and Dreams Foundation	973-361-7366
Children's Wish Foundation International	800-323-9474
Clark Health Care Products	888-895-2110
Coalition of Child Life and Therapeutic Recreation Professionals	813-893-6265
Colours in Motion Sports Chairs	800-347-4537
Columbia Medical/Bath Equipment/Car Seats	800-454-6612
Convaid Strollers	800-552-1020
Cosco	800-544-1108
Council for Exceptional Children	888-232-7733
Creative Mobility Bikes	800-711-2453
Creative Mobility Vans	619-474-4072
Creepster Crawler	800-577-1317
CycleTote Bike Trailer	800-747-2407
Daimler/Chrysler Automobility Program	800-255-9877

Dana Douglas Walkers	613-723-6734
Davis Made/Standing Dani	810-742-0581
Digisplint	519-235-2981
Disability Rights Education and Defense Fund	510-644-2555
Disability Travel and Recreation Resources	800-846-4537
Disabled Children's Relief Fund	516-377-1605
Dream Ride Car Seat/Car Bed	800-544-1108
Dreamtime Baby	866-376-8463
Drug Store Online	800-378-4786
Dynavox/Sunrise Medical	800-333-4000
Easter Seals	800-221-6827
EasyStand Standers	800-342-8968
Education Resource Information Center	800-538-3742
Efix Wheelchair Stair Climber	888-426-8581
Elks Clubs of the United States	773-755-4700
Emerging Horizons Accessible Travel News	209-599-9409
Enabling Device Toys	800-832-8697
Equipment Shop	800-525-7681
Evenflo Company	800-233-5921 (US)
	937-773-3971 (Canada)
Everest & Jennings Wheelchairs	800-235-4661
Exceptional Parent Magazine	877-372-7368
EZ-On Vest	800-323-6598
Family Voices	888-835-5669
Finally It Fits	866-866-9740
First Hand Foundation	816-201-1569
Fisher-Price	800-432-5437
Flag House Supplies	800-793-7900
Ford Motor Company	800-952-2248
Frank Mobility Systems	888-426-8581
Freedom Concept Bikes	800-661-9915
Freedom Designs	800-331-8551
Freedom Driving Aids	888-605-9999
Freedom Ryder Bikes	800-800-5828
Garaventa	800-663-6556
General Motors Assistance Program	800-323-9935

Genetic Alliance	202-966-5557
Genetic Information and Patient Services	480-539-6063
Graco Car Seats	800-345-4109 (US)
	800-667-8184 (Canada)
Granstand Standing Systems	800-827-8263
Grant a Wish Children's Promise Foundation	800-933-5470
Grants and Related Resources	517-432-6123
Guardian	800-333-4000
Hard Manufacturing	800-873-4273
Hearing Health Magazine	800-829-5934
HEATH Resource Center	800-544-3284
Hertz Supply/Volker Beds	800-321-4240
Horcher Lifting Systems	800-582-8732
Hospitals and Related Institutions	703-684-1355
Hoyer/Guardian	800-333-4000
Independence Technology Power Wheelchairs	877-794-3125
Independent Mobility Systems	800-467-8267
Infinitec Driving/Equipment Resources	312-368-0380
Innovative Products Scooters	800-950-5185
International Bone and Mineral Society	202-367-1121
Invacare Wheelchairs/Beds	800-333-6900
Jaycees	800-529-2337
Johnson & Johnson/Independence Technology I-Glide	877-794-4583
Kaye Products	919-732-6444
Kettler International Tricycles	757-427-2400
Kid-EZB Transit Model/Sunrise	888-333-2572
Kiwanis International	317-875-8755
Leisure Lift	800-255-0285
Levo Wheelchairs	888-538-6872
Lightning Hand Cycles	805-736-0700
Lions Clubs International	630-571-5466
Lite Gait Treadmill/Un-weighting System	800-332-9255
Little People of America	888-472-2001
Little Tyke Central Toys	800-321-0183
Lubidet USA	800-582-4338
Lumex/Medical Supplies Plus	800-794-8383

Maclaren USA	877-442-4622
Make a Wish Foundation	800-722-9474
March of Dimes	888-663-4637
Med Group Medical Supplies	800-825-5633
Medi-Man Lifts	800-868-0441
MedTrade Show	800-933-8735
Michigan Assistive Technology Resource	800-274-7426
Midwest Mobility Design	847-923-9892
Motion Concepts Wheelchairs/Modifications	888-433-6818
Moto Med/Great Lakes Medical	708-386-6501
Mulholland/Growth Guidance	805-525-7165
Multi-Lift/Access Unlimited	800-849-2143
My Pool Pal Flotation Swimwear	800-715-9415
National Association for the Education of Young Children	800-424-2460
National Association of Children's Hospitals and Related Institutions	703-684-1355
National Association of Protection and Advocacy Systems	202-408-9514
National Center on Accessibility	812-856-4422
National Center on Physical Activity and Disability	800-900-8086
National Clearinghouse on Postsecondary Education	800-554-3284
National Family Caregivers Association	800-896-3650
National Health Information Center	800-336-4797
National Information Center for Children and Youth with Disabilities	800-695-0285
National Institute of Child Health and Human Development	800-370-2943
National Institutes of Health	301-496-4000
National Library of Medicine	888-346-3656
National Library Services for the Blind and Handicapped	202-707-5100
National Organization for Rare Disorders	203-744-0100
National Osteoporosis Foundation	202-223-2226
National Recreation and Park Association	703-858-0784
National Rehabilitation Information Center	800-346-2742
National Resource Center on Supportive Housing and Home Modifications	213-740-1364
Natural Access Beach Wheelchairs	800-411-7789

North Coast Supplies	800-821-9319
Office of Special Education and Rehabilitative Services	202-245-7468
Open World Magazine	212-447-7284
Ortho Kinetics	800-558-7786
Osteogenesis Imperfecta Foundation	**800-981-2663**
Otto Bock Seating and Wheelchair Accessories	800-328-4058
Palaestra Magazine	309-833-1902
Paralympic Games	719-866-2030
Paralyzed Veterans of America	800-444-0120
Parent Training and Information Centers	800-695-0285
Paws With a Cause	800-253-7297
Peg Perego	800-671-1701
Permobil Power Wheelchairs	800-736-0925
Play With a Purpose	888-330-1826
Power Trainer Hand/Leg Cycle	800-852-6869
Prentke Romich Company/Augmentative Communication	800-262-1984
Pride Power Wheelchairs/Scooters	800-800-8586
Private Door Openers	800-549-9611
PT–Magazine of Physical Therapy	800-999-2782
Quickie Wheelchair/Kid Cart	888-333-2572
Radio Flyer Wagons	800-621-7613
Rand Scot Medical Supplies	800-322-2884
Recreatives All Terrain Vehicles	800-255-2511
Rehab and Therapy Products Review	714-998-6242
Ride-Away Handicap Equipment	888-743-3292
Rifton Equipment Bath/Gait/Standers	800-777-4244
ROHO/Crown Therapeutics	800-851-3449
Ronald McDonald House Charities	630-623-7048
Rotary International	847-866-3000
Rubbermaid Home Products	888-895-2110
Sammons Preston Rolyan Medical Supplies	800-323-5547
Saratoga Hand Cycle	800-474-4010
Shriners Hospitals for Children	800-237-5055(US) 800-361-7256 (Canada)
Snug Seat Car Seats/Strollers/Standers	800-336-7684
Society for Accessible Travel and Hospitality	212-447-7284

Southpaw Medical Supply	800-228-1698
Special Needs Advocate for Parents	888-310-9889
Sports and Spokes Magazine	888-888-2201
Sprint Aquatic Products	800-235-2156
Standing Dani Standing Devices	810-742-0581
Star Bright Children's Charities	800-315-2580
Star Car	800-463-5685
Starcraft Mobility	800-528-3769
Starlight Foundation	310-479-1212
Step 2 Children's Toys	800-347-8372
Step'n Go Cycles	800-648-7335
Sunrise Medical/Quickie Wheelchairs/Dynavox	888-333-2572
Sunshine Foundation	800-767-1976
SureHands Lifts	800-724-5305
Technical Assistance Alliance Coordinating Office	888-248-0822
The Dream Factory	800-456-7556
TherAdapt	800-261-4919
Therapeutic Recreation	304-599-6465
Therapeutic Recreation Professionals	301-881-7092
TheraPlay Bikes	800-306-6777
Texas Scottish Rite Hospital for Children	800-421-1121
Tip Top Wheelchair Lift	800-735-5958
Tub Slide Shower Chair	508-362-7498
Tuff Talker/Freedom Toughbook	800-869-8521
Tumble Forms/Sammons Preston	800-323-5547
Vantage Mobility Vans	800-348-8267
Variety Ability Toileting Systems	800-891-4514
Variety–The Children's Charity	888-852-1300
Volkswagen	800-374-8389
Walk Easy	800-441-2904
WebMD	201-703-3400
Wenzelite Walkers	800-706-9255
Wheelchair Getaways	800-642-2042
WheelchairNet	412-383-6793
World Congress and Exposition on Disabilities	877-923-3976

Appendix I. Quick Web References

Abilities Expo	www.abilitiesexpo.com
Abilities Magazine	www.enablelink.org
Ability Magazine	www.abilitymagazine.com
ABLEDATA	www.abledata.com
Access-Able Travel	www.access-able.com
Access for Disabled Americans	www.accessfordisabled.com
Access to Travel Magazine	www.access-able.com
Access Unlimited	www.accessunlimited.com
Ace Bandages	www.bd.com/elastics
Active Living Magazine	www.activelivingmagazine.com
Adaptive Mall for Children with Special Needs	www.adaptivemall.com
AliMed Medical Supplies	www.alimed.com
Alliance for Technology Access	www.ataccess.org
Alpha Smart	www2.alphasmart.com
Ambucs/Amtryke Specialty Bikes	www.ambucs.com/aamtryke.htm
American Academy of Orthopaedic Surgeons	www.aaos.org
American Academy of Pediatrics	www.aap.org
American Association of Persons with Disabilities	www.aapd-dc.org
American Camp Association	www.acacamps.org
American Dental Association	www.ada.org
American Discount Medical Supplies	www.Americandiscountmedical.com
American Health Consultants Resources	www.ahcpMedi.com
American Journal of Physical Medicine and Rehabilitation	www.amjphysmedrehab.com
American Medical Association	www.ama-assn.org
American Occupational Therapy Association	www.aota.org
American Physical Therapy Association	www.apta.org
American Society for Bone and Mineral Research	www.asbmr.org
Americans with Disabilities Act	www.usdoj.gov/crt/ada
American Therapeutic Recreation Association	www.atra-tr.org
Amigo Mobility Scooters	www.myamigo.com
Aquatech/Dolomite Bath Lifts	www.clarkehealthcare.com

Architectural and Transportation Barriers Compliance Board/US Access Board	www.access-board.gov
Arjo Bath Lifts	www.arjo.com
Association for Driver Rehabilitation Specialists	www.driver-ed.org
Association of University Centers on Disabilities	www.aucd.org
Athletes Helping Athletes	www.roadrunnersports.com
Baby Abby	www.babyabby.com
Barrier Free Lifts	www.barrierfreelifts.com
Benik Vests/Supports	www.benik.com
BESI Restraining Harness	www.besi-inc.com
Bike Rack Specialty Bikes	www.thebikerack.com
Biomechanics Magazine	www.cmp.com
Blaze Sports Clubs of America	www.blazesports.com
Boppy	www.boppy.com
Braun	www.braunlift.com
***Breakthrough* (OI Foundation Newsletter)**	**www.oif.org**
Britax Car Seats	www.britaxusa.com
Bruno	www.bruno.com
Canine Companions	www.caninecompanions.org
Cardon Rehabilitation Products	www.cardonrehab.com
Care Medical Supply Catalog	www.carecatalogservices.com
Careers and the disAbled Magazine	www.eop.com
Carrie Car Seat	www.tumbleforms.com
Cascade DAFO Orthoses	www.dafo.com
CDC Health Related Hoaxes	www.cdc.gov/hoax_rumors.htm
Center for Universal Design	www.design.ncsu.edu/cud
Centers for Disease Control	www.cdc.gov
Challenge Magazine	www.dsusa.org
Children's Defense Fund	www.childrensdefense.org
Children's Hopes and Dreams Foundation	www.childrenswishes.org
Children's Hospital of Philadelphia	www.chop.edu
Children's Wish Foundation International	www.childrenswish.org
Clark Health Care Products	www.clarkhealthcare.com
Clinical Trials	www.clinicaltrials.gov
Coalition of Child Life and Therapeutic Recreation Professionals	www.childlife.org

Cochrane Collaboration Medical Resources Online	www.cochrane.org
Colours in Motion	www.colourswheelchair.com
Columbia Medical	www.columbiamedical.com
Convaid	www.convaid.com
Cosco	www.coscojuvenile.com
Council for Exceptional Children	www.cec.sped.org
Creative Mobility Bikes	www.creativemobility.net
Creative Mobility Vans	www.creativemobility.com
Creepster Crawler	www.redbarn-enter.com
CycleTote Bike Trailer	www.cycletote.com
Daimler/Chrysler Automobility Program	www.dc-automobility.com
Dana Douglas Walkers	www.danadouglas.com
Davis Made/Standing Dani	www.standingdani.com
Digisplint	www.digisplint.ca
Disability Resource Organization	www.disabilityresources.org
Disability Rights Education and Defense Fund	www.dredf.org
Disability Travel and Recreation Resource	www.makoa.org/travel.htm
Disabled Children's Relief Fund	www.dcrf.com
Dream Ride Car Seat/ Car Bed	www.coscojuvenile.com
Dreamtime Baby	www.dreamtimebaby.com
Dr. Koop Medical Resources	www.drkoop.com
Drug Store Online	www.drugstore.com
Dynavox/Sunrise Medical	www.sunrisemedical.com
Easter Seals	www.easterseals.com
EasyStand Standers	www.easystand.com
Education Resource Information Center	www.eric.ed.gov
Efix Wheelchair Stair Climber	www.frankmobility.com
Elks Clubs of the United States	www.elks.org
Emerging Horizons Accessible Travel News	www.emerginghorizons.com
Enabling Device Toys	www.enablingdevices.com
Equipment Shop	www.equipmentshop.com
Etac Sverige AB Wheelchairs for Sports	www.etac.net
Evenflow Company	www.evenflo.com
Exceptional Parent Magazine	www.exceptionalparent.com
EZ-On Vest	www.ezonpro.com

Family Voices	www.familyvoices.org
Finally It Fits	www.finallyitfits.com
First Hand Foundation	www.firsthandfoundation.org
Fisher-Price	www.fisher-price.com/us
Flag House Supplies	www.flaghouse.com
Ford Motor Company	www.mobilitymotoringprogram.com
Frank Mobility Systems	www.frankmobility.com
Freedom Concept Bikes	www.freedomconcepts.com
Freedom Designs	www.freedomdesigns.com
Freedom Driving Aids	www.freedomdrivingaids.com
Freedom Ryder Bikes	www.freedomryder.com
Free Medical Journals Resource Site	www.freemedicaljournals.com
Garaventa	www.garaventa.ca
General Motors Assistance Program	www.GMmobility.com
Genetic Alliance	www.geneticalliance.org
Genetic Information and Patient Services	www.icomm.ca/geneinfo
Graco Car Seats	www.gracobaby.com
Granstand Standing Systems	www.primeengineering.com
Grant a Wish Children's Promise Foundation	www.grant-a-wish.org
Grants and Related Resources	
	www.lib.msu.edu/harris23/grants/servicec.htm
Guardian	www.sunrisemedical.com
Hard Manufacturing	www.hardmfg.com
Health and Medical Information/Resources	www.healthgate.com
HealthCare Market Place Resources	www.hcmarketplace.com
Health on the Net Foundation	www.hon.ch
Hearing Health Magazine	www.hearinghealthmag.com
HEATH Resource Center	www.heath.gwu.edu
Hertz Supply/Volker Beds	www.hertzsupply.com
Hi-Ethics	www.hiethics.com
Horcher Lifting Systems	www.horcher.com
Hospitals and Related Institutions	www.childrenshospitals.net
Hoyer/Guardian Lifts	www.sunrisemedical.com
Independence Technology Power Wheelchairs	www.indetech.com
Independent Mobility Systems	www.Rampvan.net
Infinitec Driving/Equipment Resources	www.infinitec.org

Infinite Potential Through Assistive Technology	www.infinitec.org
Institute for Child Health Policy	www.ichp.edu
International Bone and Mineral Society	www.ibmsonline.org
Invacare	www.invacare.com
Jaycees	www.usjaycees.com
Johnson & Johnson I-Glide	www.ibotnow.com
Journal of Bone and Joint Surgery	www.ejbjs.org
Journal of Pediatric Orthopaedics	www.pedorthopaedics.com
Journal of the American Medical Association	www.jama.ama-assn.org
Journal of the American Occupational Therapy Association	www.aota.org/ajot/index.asp
Journal of the American Physical Therapy Association	www.ptjournal.org
Kaye Products	www.Kayeproducts.com
Kettler Tricycles	www.Kettlerusa.com
Kid-EZB Transit Model/Sunrise	www.sunrisemedical.com
Kids Health Resources	www.kidshealth.org
Kiwanis International	www.kiwanis.org
Leisure Lift	www.pacesaver.com
Levo Wheelchairs	www.levousa.com
Lightning Hand Cycles	www.lightningbikes.com
Lions Clubs International	www.lionsclubs.org
Lite Gait Treadmill/Un-weighting System	www.litegait.com
Little People of America	www.LPAonline.org
Little Tyke Toys	www.littletykecentral.com
Lubidet	www.lubidet.com
Lumex Medical Supplies Plus	www.medicalsuppliesplus.com
Maclaren USA	www.maclarenbaby.com
Mainstream Magazine	www.mainstream-mag.com
Make a Wish Foundation	www.wish.org
March of Dimes	www.modimes.org
Med Group Medical Supplies	www.medrehab.net
Medi-Man Lifts	www.medi-man.com
MedlinePlus	www.medlineplus.gov
Medscape WebMD Health Information	www.medscape.com
Med Source Consulting Groups	www.medsource.com

Med Trade Show	www.medtrade.com
Merck Manual Online Resource	www.merck.com/pubs
Michigan Assistive Technology Resource	www.cenmi.org/matr/aboutus.asp
Motion Concepts Wheelchairs/Modifications	www.motionconcepts.com
Moto Med/Great Lakes Medical	www.greatlakesmedical.com
Mulholland/Growth Guidance	www.mulhollandinc.com
Multi-Lift/Access Unlimited	www.accessunlimited.com
My Pool Pal Flotation Swimwear	www.mypoolpal.com
National Association for the Education of Young Children	www.naeyc.org
National Association of Children's Hospitals and Related Institutions	www.childrenshospitals.net
National Association of Protection and Advocacy Systems	www.napas.org
National Center on Accessibility	www.indiana.edu/~nca/
National Center on Physical Activity and Disability	www.ncpad.org
National Clearinghouse on Postsecondary Education	www.heath.gwu.edu
National Early Childhood Technical Assistance Center	www.nectas.unc.edu
National Family Caregivers Association	www.nfcacares.org
National Health Information Center	www.healthgov/nhic
National Information Center for Children and Youth with Disabilities	www.nichcy.org
National Institute of Child Health and Human Development	www.nichd.nih.gov
National Institutes of Health	www.nih.gov
National Library of Medicine	www.nlm.nih.gov
National Organization for Rare Disorders	www.rarediseases.org
National Osteoporosis Foundation	www.nof.org
National Recreation and Park Association	www.nrpa.org
National Rehabilitation Information Center	www.naric.com
National Resource Center on Supportive Housing and Home Modifications	www.homemods.org
Natural Access Beach Wheelchairs	www.landeez.com
Nemours Children's Programs	www.nemours.org

New England Journal of Medicine	www.nejm.org
New Mobility Magazine	www.newmobility.com
North Coast Supplies	www.northcoastmedical.com
Office of Special Education and Rehabilitative Services	www.ed.gov/offices/OSERS
Open World Magazine	www.sath.org
Ortho Kinetics	www.ez-international.com
Osteogenesis Imperfecta Foundation	**www.oif.org**
Osteogenesis Imperfecta Federation of Europe	www.oife.org
Otto Bock Seating and Wheelchair Accessories	www.ottobockus.com
Palaestra Magazine	www.palaestra.com
Paralympic Games	www.usparalympics.org
Paralyzed Veterans of America	www.pva.org
Parent Training and Information Centers	www.TaAlliance.org/centers
Paws With a Cause	www.pawswithacause.org
Peg Perego	www.perego.com
Permobil Power Wheelchairs	www.permobilusa.com
Play With a Purpose	www.playwithapurpose.com
Power Trainer Hand/Leg Cycle	www.scifit.com
Prentke Romich Company/Augmentative Communication	www.prentrom.com
Pride Power Wheelchairs/Scooters	www.pridemobility.com
Private Door Openers	www.privatedoor.com
PT–Magazine of Physical Therapy	www.apta.org
PubMed Journal Articles	www.ncbi.nih.gov/entrez/query.fcgi
PubMed Resources	www.pubmed.gov
Quickie Wheelchair/Kid Cart	www.sunrisemedical.com
Radio Flyer Wagons	www.radioflyer.com
Rand Scot Medical Supplies	www.riconcorp.com
Rehab and Therapy Products Review	www.rtproductsreview.com
Ride-Away Equipment	www.ride-away.com
Rifton Equipment	www.rifton.com
ROHO/Crown Therapertics	www.therohogroup.com
Ronald McDonald House Charities	www.rmhc.com
Rotary Clubs International	www.rotary.org
Rubbermaid Home Products	www.rubbermaid.com

Sammons Preston Rolyan	www.sammonspreston.com
Saratoga Hand Cycle	www.randscot.com
Shriners Hospitals for Children	www.shrinershq.org
Snug Seat Car Seats/Strollers/Standers	www.snugseat.com
Society for Accessible Travel and Hospitality	www.sath.org
Southpaw Medical Supply	www.southpawenterprises.com
Special Needs Advocate for Parents	www.snapinfo.org
Sports and Spokes Magazine	www.sns-magazine.com
Sprint Aquatic Products	www.sprintaquatics.com
Standing Dani Standing Devices	www.standingdani.com
Star Bright Children's Charities	www.starbright.org
Star Car	www.tashinc.com
Starlight Foundation	www.slsb.org
Step 2 Children's Toys	www.step2.com
Step'n Go Cycle	www.stepngo.com
Sunrise Medical/Quickie Wheelchairs	www.sunrisemedical.com
Sunshine Foundation	www.sunshinefoundation.org
SureHands Lifts	www.surehands.com
Technical Assistance Alliance Coordinating Office	www.TaAlliance.org
Texas Scottish Rite Hospital for Children	www.tsrhc.org
The Bones Page	www.geocities.com/CapeCanaveral/Lab/3608
The Dream Factory	www.dreamfactoryinc.com
TherAdapt	www.theradapt.com
Therapeutic Recreation Professionals	www.childlife.org
Therapeutic Recreation	www.recreationtherapy.com
TheraPlay Bikes	www.Triaid.com
Tip Top Wheelchair Lift	www.minot.com/~tiptop/
Tub Slide Shower Chair	www.rdequipment.com
Tuff Talker/Freedom Toughbook	www.words-plus.com
Tumble Forms/Sammons Preston	www.sammonspreston.com
Vantage Mobility Vans	www.vantagemobility.com
Variety Ability Toileting Systems	www.vasi.on.ca
Variety–The Children's Charity	www.usvariety.org
Virtual Hospital Resources	www.vh.org
Volkswagen	www.VW.com

Walk Easy	www.walkeasy.com
WebMD	www.webmd.com
Wenzelite Walkers	www.wenzelite.com
Wheelchair Getaways	www.wheelchairgetaways.com
WheelchairNet	www.wheelchairnet.org
World Congress and Exposition on Disabilities	www.wcdexpo.com

Please note that the companies, organizations, Web sites, search engines, products, and services listed above are for reference and information purposes only and do not constitute an endorsement.

Additional Resources
from the OI Foundation

Therapeutic Strategies for OI:
A Guide for Physical and Occupational Therapists *(booklet)*
This 14-page photo-illustrated booklet is intended for medical professionals or for families to use as a resource while working with a medical professional. The book is compiled from information from PTs, OTs, and physicians familiar with OI. It includes information about the disorder, the role of physical and occupational therapy in managing OI, safe handling of children and adults with OI, and specific strategies for safe, successful therapy for people with OI.
　　　Price: FREE (single copies)

Growing Up with OI:
A Guide for Families & Caregivers *(book)*
Addresses the most common questions parents, family members, and caregivers have about raising a child with OI. The focus is on maximizing a child's abilities and proactive problem solving. The book covers the medical aspects of OI, as well as the emotional, financial, and relationship challenges that families living with OI face. Chapters are written by people with OI, their parents, and medical professionals.

Growing Up with OI:
A Guide for Children *(book)*
Written especially for elementary school-aged children, this book focuses on the same issues as the adult version. It encourages children to focus on their strengths and abilities and provides problem-solving advice for challenges they may face.
　　　Price: $10 each; or both "Growing Up" books for $17

OI: A Guide for Nurses *(book)*
This 64-page book is a comprehensive guide to assist nursing professionals as they come into contact with patients with osteogenesis imperfecta. Written, edited, and reviewed by more than twenty nurses, nurse practitioners, and medical professionals with extensive OI experience, this book offers practical insight into diagnosis, family education, standard treatments, medical procedures, and care for patients of all ages—and much, much more. It is intended for nursing professionals and nursing students, or for families to provide as a resource when working with nursing professionals unfamiliar with OI.
　　　Price: FREE (single copies)

Jason's First Day *(children's book and educator's guide)*
This picture book tells the story of the first day of school for a child with OI. It is designed to be read to preschool, kindergarten, and first grade children. The book includes a teacher's guide and resources for educators to make the transition to school easier for children with OI or other mobility impairing disabilities.
> Price: $8.50

Caring for Infants and Children with OI *(booklet)*
Covers the basics of caring for a child with OI from birth to 3 years old. It includes specific examples and advice regarding handling, adaptive equipment, medical treatments, education, and the emotional issues involved in raising a child with OI. One of the Foundation's most popular resources, it is a companion to the video *You Are Not Alone*. (Also available in Spanish.)
> Price: FREE (1-5 copies)

Fact Sheets and Other Resources
The OI Foundation has a number of fact sheets, videos, and other resources, most of them available free of charge. For a complete list, visit our Web site at www.oif.org, or contact our Information On Demand service and ask for a resource list.

Information On Demand
Information resource specialists are available from 9 a.m. to 5 p.m. Monday through Friday to respond to your specific questions about OI with medically verified information. They can also provide you with information about specialists familiar with OI and assist you in finding peer support through local networking groups or support volunteers.

Call 800-981-2663 or e-mail bonelink@oif.org to speak with an information resource specialist.

Ordering Printed Resources
To order resources from the Foundation, visit www.oif.org, call 800-981-2663, or request the resource by title (and enclose a check, if applicable) by writing to:

> Osteogenesis Imperfecta Foundation, Inc.
> 800 West Diamond Avenue, Suite 210
> Gaithersburg, MD 20878

About the OI Foundation

The Osteogenesis Imperfecta Foundation was founded in 1970 when a group of parents of children with OI joined together to provide mutual support, enhance public and professional awareness of OI, and promote research. The Foundation's original purpose continues to shape our vision: funding research to find treatments and a cure, and providing support to help people with OI and their families cope with daily life. The mission of the Osteogenesis Imperfecta Foundation, Inc., is to improve the quality of life for people with osteogenesis imperfecta through education, increasing awareness, encouraging mutual support, and promoting research to find treatments and a cure.

How the OI Foundation Helps

People with OI can and do live satisfying and successful lives. Like other children, those with OI attend school, make friends, go on family vacations, and participate in sports. Like other adults, those with OI earn advanced degrees, socialize with friends, build careers, marry, and have families. Those living with OI also face daily challenges because of their bone disorder. The OI Foundation helps people with OI face those challenges and improve their lives through information, support, research, education, and awareness.

Information

The OI Foundation provides information resources to educate people about this bone disorder. The OI Foundation has answers for parents just learning about their child's OI diagnosis, adults grappling with the lifelong medical problems associated with OI, and medical professionals seeking information to improve treatment for their patients. Information resources include *Breakthrough*, a free quarterly newsletter, as well as an informative Web site, monthly electronic news bulletins, fact sheets, brochures, videos, audiocassettes, and books. The Foundation also provides individual responses to every inquiry with medically verified information.

Support

Through a network of volunteer-run support and networking groups and support volunteers, the Foundation connects people in need with people who can share similar experiences, coping techniques, and resources. An online chat room is available through the Foundation's Web site at www.oif.org. A biennial national conference draws hundreds of people affected by OI together for several days of learning and support.

Research

The OI Foundation provides grants for research into the causes and treatments of OI, as well as postdoctoral fellowships to attract promising new scientists to OI research. The Foundation is developing Linked Clinical Research Centers to improve the quality of care for people with OI and facilitate research progress. The Foundation also coordinates scientific workshops that focus attention on solving research problems and developing new areas of study.

Education and Awareness

Because OI is rare, many people are unfamiliar with the disorder. Even many medical, educational, and social services professionals—those whom people with OI rely on for assistance—look for opportunities to expand their knowledge of OI. The Foundation enhances public and professional awareness of OI through professional conferences, medical education resources, and media relations.

Contact the OI Foundation

The Osteogenesis Imperfecta Foundation welcomes all inquiries and provides opportunities for volunteers with an interest in helping the Foundation fulfill its mission. Learn more about the Foundation by visiting our Web site at www.oif.org, calling the Foundation at 800-981-2663, or writing to us at:

Osteogenesis Imperfecta Foundation, Inc.
804 West Diamond Avenue, Suite 210
Gaithersburg, MD 20878